Brushing Away The Tears

By Debbie Wilson

Bellissima Publishing, LLC
Jamul, California
www.bellissimapublishing.com

Copyright © 2009 by Bellissima Publishing, LLC

All rights reserved. No part of this book may be reproduced or transmitted in any form or by any means, electronic or mechanical, including any photocopying, or recording, or by any information or storage retrieval system, without permission from the publisher and author.

IBSN 1-935118-76-5
First Edition

For Christopher

Introduction

"Brushing Away the Tears" paints a portrait of a life lived with and taken by AIDS. It is the true story of Christopher Colt's journey through HIV/AIDS, and it is told in his own words, through his journals and letters, and through the journals and letters of his mother. The entries begin in 1989 when Christopher was diagnosed with HIV and ends a few months before his death in 1992 at age 39. A budding artist, Christopher details the heartbreaking fear of knowing that his time is limited and that his life is more than likely coming to an end. The footnote narrative is provided by Christopher's sister, Debbie Wilson, who holds a BA in journalism.

The subject of AIDS has been written about numerous times from a medical standpoint, but few times from the victim's view. *"Brushing Away the Tears,"* written in these firsthand accounts, stimulates the curiosity of those who wish to probe the very personal side of coping with a terminal illness.

Christopher was a radiant star whose spirit lives on through his art and whose story will inspire others to "live like you are dying."

This book speaks to the social stigma of AIDS without preaching or malice and seeks to put a face on AIDS. The face is that of a man in the prime of his life, someone who is loved by his family and who has friends and colleagues. His story is tragic, but in the midst of the narrative of terrible physical pain and tremendous fear, there is humor in the writing and in the business of everyday living.

The title *"Brushing Away the Tears"* is derived from Christopher's passion as an artist. Every life is painted with the artistic hand of God, and Christopher's life was no different. He just lived his life differently, and sometimes difference is good, especially if that difference is family and love.

Brushing Away The Tears

By Debbie Wilson

Brushing Away The Tears

8/23/92

Dear Mom,

If you open this before I get there, please try to look upon these journals as a gift, even though it is a very painful gift right now. I try to remember that Christopher would want us to smile as we hear his voice in his writings. I suggest you start with 1989 or 1990. The last two journals are full of his pain – although there is ever-lasting belief and hope that he would get better. Whatever, they are a wonderful reminder of what a special person Christopher was; and we can all be so proud of the loving, strong person he became.

Love, Debbie

Mom's Journal Entries

Friday, May 5th 1989*

Bad news. Deb called. Christopher is in the hospital. Spinal meningitis, but not confirmed. Tested him for AIDS, but it will be first of next week before we hear. Sat by the phone all day. I'm so worried. Talked to Deb many times today.

Saturday, May 6, 1989

Deb called, still no good news. Help me God, I need your help now.

Sunday, May 7, 1989

Talked to Deb and Christopher. He seems OK, but still no results.

Monday, May 8, 1989

So worried about Christopher. Still haven't heard from Donnie's test. I fear the worst.

Tuesday, May 9, 1990

Deb called before I left for school. So depressed. I can't knock the feeling of the worst from Los Angeles . I went to Wal-mart and the grocery store early. Deb has called 3 times today, and it's only 2 p.m. I think she's not telling me the bad news.

**Footnotes (what I have to say)

My mom, Hazel Wilson, also kept a journal for as long as I can remember and always encouraged me to do so as well. My brother, Christopher, was born as Donald Steven Wilson, and in the course of career changes, etc. decided to use the "also known as" Christopher Colt. It was harder for the family in Alabama to get used to the Christopher, so you will see in some of Mom's journal entries, him referred to as Donnie.

As I sit here in the El Matador Beach parking lot, so many memories come flooding back to me, memories of Christopher. I can almost hear his laughter as we walked down the rocky, steep path to the magnificent beach. He was always watchful of me---the big brother taking care of his little sister. The climb down was always punctuated with photo ops. Such a beautiful beach! We would either lie on the beach or walk along the rocky shoreline, sitting on rocks, talking or wading in the cold Pacific Ocean. Christopher never failed to honor my request to go to the beach when I visited him in Los Angeles. My first visit was in June of 1983 with my parents. Christopher drove me to Santa Monica Beach. Even though it was June, temperatures were in the 60s on the beach, so my hopes of working on a Pacific Coast tan were dashed. The people watching opportunities were plentiful!

Through the years I would visit him every year or so until I tried the job market in 1988. For a few months I was a "temp" at a bank. Christopher drove me to work every day for two months and threw me a wonderful birthday party during my stay that fall. Birthdays and holidays were a big deal to him, and he worked hard to ensure the honoree was king or queen for the entire day. He shopped for months for just the right present. His last grand shopping spree was for my 32nd birthday.

Western Union Mailgram to Mom from Christopher 3/1/81

ON THIS YOUR BIRTHDAY I REJOICE WITH YOU AND THANK YOU FOR THE GIFT OF LIFE YOU GAVE ME. ALL THAT I AM, I AM BECAUSE OF YOU. I LOVE YOU DEEPLY, FULLY FROM THE DEPTHS OF MY HEART. HAPPY BIRTHDAY, MOTHER.

Brushing Away The Tears

Matthew's Speech

From Matthew's (Christopher's partner's) speech at Christopher's memorial service in January of 1993 in Los Angeles:

"Ultimately, I believe that joy and gratitude were at the core of Christopher's character, and form the cornerstone of his legacy to us. No one who ever worked, traveled, painted or went shopping with Christopher could fail to detect an extra spark about him, a special zest that entranced me from the moment I met him. And the scary but delightful truth is, he was like that almost all the time!"

**Footnote - I eventually moved to Los Angeles, arriving on April Fools' day 1989. My arrival date seems appropriate now that I look back on what was to come.

My Mom and I had a wonderful journey across the country stopping at popular tourist spots and driving for a time along Route 66. Slices of Americana. I was sad to be moving so far away from home, as family has always been important to me. But I was glad to be closer to my big brother and the promise of more career opportunities. I lived with him and his partner, Matthew, for a while until my roommates from Nashville arrived.

It was 1989 and interesting job opportunities had dried up in Nashville. My roommates, Jeff and Brian, and I were ready for adventure and ready to try life on the west coast. Since I had secretarial skills that could gain me immediate employment with a temp agency, and I had a place to stay, it was determined that I would go to Los Angeles ahead of Jeff and Brian.

I introduced Matthew to my brother when we were working at a local radio station together in 1986. I was employed as a radio news reporter, and Matthew was a disc jockey. We worked for the "hot" station in town, and it was owned by rock and roller Sam Phillips of Sun Records fame. Mr. Phillips and his managers enjoyed outrageous promotions, and Matthew was their most dynamic DJ. He was often required to wear a tuxedo when he was broadcasting live from a business. I was having a party at my apartment in honor of Christopher's Christmas visit home, and Matthew attended wearing his tux as he had just completed a live broadcast. Christopher was enchanted with his attire not realizing that the everyday attire of a disc jockey is far from formal wear! Matthew and Christopher were smitten from the moment they met. My co-workers at the radio station immediately noticed the transformation in Matthew. Previously, he was unhappy in his personal life and with his career. Suddenly, through Christopher's eyes, he was a new man with a new destiny.

7

Brushing Away The Tears

Three years later, I was ready for a new destiny. Although the promise of adventure and more varied career opportunities were my primary motivation for moving 2,000 miles, there was also a nagging feeling that something stronger than career was pulling me to the "City of Angels." I had barely been in L.A. a month when, at the age of 29, my whole world came crashing down.

I was getting dressed for work on Cinco de Mayo, 1989, when Matthew and I heard a loud thumping sound from the shower where my brother was. Matthew discovered Christopher beating his head against the shower walls – uncontrollably it turned out. We rushed him to the emergency room and were told because of his uninsured status we would have to take him to Harbor Medical Center, a UCLA research hospital and also known as "county hospital."

We were given the devastating news that he was HIV positive a few days after his admission to the hospital. He was strong for us, and we tried to be strong for him. At first, he didn't want me to tell my parents and for several days. I didn't. The fear and loneliness I felt at being so far away from the rest of my family finally found me making the call. I tried to be strong for them and downplay the intensity of the fear and pain we felt. Instead, I tried to focus on hope and medical advances. I also assured them how Christopher, along with his partner and the small group of friends that would know this terrible news, would do everything to fight the cruel disease.

Letter to Mom from Christopher, April 11, 1988

Dear Mom:

I don't mean to write bad news but John* died last week. 27 years old and he had completed school. It was so sad. This AIDS thing is very serious and even more serious in San Francisco. I'm so thankful for my relationship with Matthew. Relationships are definitely in now. I don't think John's death has really hit me yet, but I try not to think about it much. The last time I saw him, I knew he didn't have long and couldn't bear to even call him for fear he had died. Thank God I did call before he died. The last time I was there his mother left the room immediately when I came in. I was totally unable to believe that even under those circumstances people can't let go of their prejudices.

**Footnote - John had been Christopher's lover several years earlier in the pre-AIDS days. John was also from Alabama and the two of them had moved to California together.

Mom's Journal Entery

Brushing Away The Tears

May 10, 1989

I feel so much better today after learning the results of Donnie's test. Still sad news, but not what we expected. Donnie called late. *

Author's note

*We were telling them only that it was spinal meningitis at first – should I delete the above entry by Mom to avoid confusion?

Despite the half- truths we were telling her during the first several days of his hospitalization, she knew that things were not going well.

Mom's Journal Entries

May 12, 1989

I'm so depressed. Can't shake off this sad feeling.

May 14th, 1989

Rainy. Talked to Deb and Donnie. They got me flowers for Mother's Day. My Mom is at her sister's, and I missed seeing her today.

**Footnote - Mom was also caring for her mother, who had leukemia and was in the early stages of Alzheimer's disease. My grandmother lived alone, next door to my parents as my grandfather had passed away in 1986. One of Mom's two brothers was diagnosed with brain cancer in 1991 and passed away that same year. Her sister also lived nearby, but she didn't assist very much with my grandmother's care, especially when the symptoms of Alzheimer's became obvious. As a result, my mother was the primary caregiver for her own mother during this difficult time.

Christopher spent about a week in the hospital. It was decided that he and Matthew would travel to Alabama at the end of May for Memorial Day. Understandably, Mom and Dad were anxious to see him, and he was equally anxious to assure them that he was fine. I stayed behind in Los Angeles, because I couldn't afford the trip.

We all settled into a routine of avoiding the subject of AIDS and adjusted to Christopher's ritual of doctors and lots of medicines. Christopher drank lots of water, exercised, and ate healthier. He painted with the passion of someone who knew their time was limited, focusing tremendous energy on his painting and channeling his fears into his art. Christopher also poured his anxious feelings into his journals.

In putting together the amazing story of the last years of my brother's life, I have included excerpts from his journals, as well as family letters, in hopes of communicating the depth of his fear and pain. In the first year after the frightening news of his HIV status, the journals detailed more about his struggle to become an artist than information about his physical woes. As he became increasingly ill, the journals reflected his growing concern about the possibility of dying as well as his frustration about his numerous health issues.

Christopher, as well as I, kept journals from a very young age. He began to word process his journals when he obtained employment with a large Los Angeles law firm and was able to incorporate his journals into his learning routine. The journal entries not only detailed his struggle with his art, but also revealed his sense of humor. I am so grateful that he left such wonderful documents of his life.

Monday, Nov. 20, 1989

It's almost time to go home. I'm kind of feeling sick to my stomach. I hope it passes. I guess I'll go to group therapy tonight. I have so much to do. I must not procrastinate. I hope this is how one spells procrastinate.

I'm at an impasse with my art right now. Can I paint? That is the question. It's that damn border project. It's wigging me out. I don't like it. I should probably start it over. It only takes something like that project to really bum me out. Oh well.

There is a terrible flu virus going around. I hope I don't get it. I pray to God I don't get it!

Letter to Christopher from Mom

November 30, 1989

Dear Donnie:

I'm so sorry about your latest art disaster, but shucks, that happens to every great person. Just ask Van Gogh or Rembrandt. Worse things probably happened to them. You really have to bounce back and probably do it better the 2nd time. Any how, I'm sorry.

**Footnote - Christopher did not often talk about his religious beliefs. As a youngster in the small southern town of Florence, Alabama, he attended church regularly. Growing up he disliked organized religion intensely. He continued, however, to worship God in his private way and often mentioned prayer in his journal entries.

His writings echo the frustrations artists of varied disciplines often feel when confronted with the chores of everyday living, chores that keep artists from doing what they love the most. It became especially frustrating for Christopher because he knew deep down inside that he did not have the years of tomorrows that most people take for granted. His list of "things to do before I die" became more important. High on that list was his desire of creating art that would earn him the coveted title of artist.

Tuesday, November 21, 1989

What to say. I haven't been painting at all. I went to group last night. It was interesting to say the least. Back to the painting. It seems like there are a lot of household chores to do. Tonight we have to go shopping. Is this an excuse to not paint? First and foremost do I want to paint? I'm at an impasse right now for sure. I'm kind of intimidated by it all. This is hard to explain in words. It's that damn border project again. I want to paint so bad that the need overshadows my ability to perform. Does that make any sense? I wonder. Anyway, I shall overcome.

I'm just reading over the text of this journal and I realized that I don't have to do anything that I don't want to do. I wrote that I have to go shopping. Well, I don't have to. I must want to. This all sounds very intellectual again. It goes back to the same old thing about feeling like everything is a chore instead of a choice.

Thank God!!! I feel better today than I did yesterday. I felt like shit all day. Matthew has been so sweet to me. So much to do in the next few days. Thanksgiving. What do I have to give thanks for? First, Matthew, then my family, then my health for what it is, and my art. I really have a lot to be thankful for. I didn't mean to make this corny. Anyway, that's the way it was, Tuesday, November 21, 1989.

Monday, Nov. 26th, 1989

I'm feeling fine today. Nowadays that is a good sign. I hate those days when I feel like shit. Excuse the language.

I still didn't finalize my masterpiece project. I just can't make up my mind about that damn project. Why? Because I'm stupid? I don't think so. I feel I can be a great artist if given the opportunity. What opportunity is that, you ask? The opportunity to learn. The opportunity to get out of my own way.

I've decided what I'm going to do for the top of my border project. Yea!!! Anyway, I hope it goes well. You know I started it over. I just wasn't pleased with the first attempt. I want to paint!!!!! More than that I want to paint well. I want to know what I am doing. Oh God, please use me as your instrument or brush or whatever. This is beginning to sound corny. I don't care. I love art. I love art. Oh

God, I'm excited. I hope I live long enough to see my studies finished. You know what I mean?

I'm still reading the Van Gogh biography. I love it, I love it, I love it! I think it's inspirational.

Tuesday, November 28, 1989

Last night I did almost finish that border project. It looks OK. Just a little tidying up and bingo it will be done. Now, on to the next project. I've decided not to get uptight about this analysis project.

I'm not feeling as well as I did yesterday. I think I'm trying to get the flu. I sure hope not. It could prove to be fatal in my case. I'm not going to expound on this.

**Footnote - I always knew Christopher was a protective big brother. I didn't find out how alarmed he was about my desire to go skydiving until I was reading some of his old letters to our Mom that I found while writing this book.

Letter To Mom From Christopher

December 1, 1989

Dear Mom:

Talked to Deb a few minutes ago. She said that Jeff called me last night to talk with me about her Christmas present. He actually talked to Matthew. They, (Jeff and Bryan – my roommates) want to give her a certificate good for, now get this, a parachute jump, complete with pictures while in the air! I think this is too dangerous, but you know Deb. They say she wants to do it. I don't think it's a good idea. What do you think? They want my advice. I'm going to try and stall them if possible. I need your input. Please advise.

Tell everyone I said hi and that I'm looking forward to seeing everybody. I love all of you so very much. You'll never know how much it means having a family like ours. We are all truly lucky to have each other.

P.S. 3 weeks until Christmas!!!

Monday, December 4, 1989

I had a strange weekend. I was sick Friday and Saturday. Had to miss my class. I feel a little guilty in that I wasn't totally prepared for class. Did I use being ill as part of an excuse not to go? I wonder. I'm not really sure. Deb said it was more important for me to get my rest. Perhaps.

Tuesday, December 5, 1989

Brushing Away The Tears

The day is wearing on. Had an intense discussion with Kurt* last night over treatment. The main discussion was am I doing enough? Is working that important? I don't know what else to do. I guess I could be doing more than I am. It's time to make major decisions. I do feel sick right now. I think I do have the flu. Maureen* said that it is possible to get the flu just like everyone else. I don't think it is time to panic. Concerned yes, panicked no. I've just got to keep myself healthy for the time being.

Footnotes:
*Kurt was an HIV+ patient in Christopher's support therapy group.
*Maureen was one of the nurse practitioners at UCLA Harbor Medical Center.

Now for other matters at hand. I didn't work on my project last night. Why? I was not only tired, but kind of at a loss as to what I'm supposed to be doing. I guess it's all in the name of art and learning. I do want to learn how to paint. I wonder if I ever will.

I'm beginning to panic a little over this health problem. I think I'm beginning to wonder if I'm going to be all right. It keeps coming back to that. I guess Kurt scared me a little. It seems to me that he was a little self-righteous. I need some professional help on this matter.

Footnote - The first year Christopher complained very little and said little about his health or AIDS. We all tip-toed around these issues, even though I constantly encouraged him to get plenty of rest. I sometimes wondered if he would be better off quitting his job to concentrate on his health. Ultimately, his personality dictated that things remain as normal as possible. Christopher was raised in the South with a strong work ethic; and despite some challenging years of rebellious activities, he always worked and earned his living. It was *not* in his nature to be lazy or self-pitying.

Monday, December 11, 1989

It's Monday again. I've got a lot to do this week! Clinic. Boo hiss! I hope all goes well. We'll see. I guess I'm almost over the flu. Who knows how I feel these days. I know I don't.

Monday, December 18, 1989

I hope I can work it out where I have a career in the arts. It really would be nice if I could go back to school and finish my degree. I know what I want to do for a living. It took long enough!!! I know I want to do something in the art field. Still, I don't know just what.

My Writing

It was always exciting for Christopher to return home to rural Alabama. At his request, few people knew he had AIDS. Christopher feared that his brothers and others in the community might not want him to be around them or their children if they knew he had AIDS. One has to remember that the subject of AIDS was not widely discussed in small towns like Florence, Alabama.

For Christmas 1989, both Christopher and I flew home to be with our family and friends.

Tuesday December 19th, 1989

The time for our departure is getting close. Am I prepared? How does one prepare to go home? It's never like I envision it to be. I've learned to just roll with the punches. Hopefully, it will be fun. I hope I can get some painting done while I'm there. We shall see. It would be sad to lug all those supplies home and not do anything with them. So I shall do my best to PAINT.

I'm going shopping tonight with Renee. I hope we have shopper's karma! Shopping Karma!!!!!!!

Mom's Journal Entries

Saturday, December 23, 1989

Went to the grocery store to get ready for Donnie and Matthew's arrival. They arrived at 2:30 a.m. Cooked a big breakfast. Matthew ate with us before leaving for his parent's house. Everyone was in and out all day and the phone ringing constantly.

Monday, December 25, 1989

White Christmas!

Christopher's Journal Entries

Monday, December 25, 1989

Well, it's Christmas and I'm at Mom and Dad's. We're getting ready for Christmas dinner. It snowed here last night so we had a white Christmas. I've got to paint at least once. Hopefully I will have the chance to do it some more. Actually, it is harder to find the time here. There have been so many people here that it is hard to find the time to do anything but visit. It's nice but I need to paint soon or I shall go crazy.

People have started to arrive for dinner. Glenn and Teresa that is. I guess I should get out there and visit with them. I'm truly lucky to have such a wonderful family. I am truly lucky to have gotten this typewriter from Katy's house. I love to type! It's Christmas time at Grandma's house.

Tuesday, December 26, 1989

Well, it's one day after Christmas and Deb and I are going to meet Matthew. Teresa just left with the kids. Those kids are so loud!!! I love it!! Still haven't painted yet. Maybe I will and maybe I won't. I would like to go to Cajuns and have oysters on the half shell. I would like to do some walking around, maybe some driving around. Matthew is here. B.F.D. Yo Mama.

The times Christopher and I spent together in Alabama were so special to me. We shared the guest bedroom in twin beds. Even in adulthood, he was always the first to wake up Christmas morning and he had a way of renewing the sense of wonder and excitement of Santa Claus!

By the end of the 80s, AIDS had spread rapidly and the media routinely covered it. There were reminders everywhere.

Christopher's Journal Entry

Wednesday, December 27th, 1989

As Mom, Dad and I watched a show tonight about the 80s, I became very uneasy, as I knew it would get to a segment on AIDS. Indeed they did and I was <u>very</u> uneasy, but I sat through it. Mom and Dad were nervous too. No one said anything, but we all endured it. We didn't learn much, but we sat through it. I think I'm kind of sick of the whole thing myself.

I was strongly influenced by Christopher to appreciate our town's attractions and beauty. When I was 10 or 12 years old he wanted to ride by a home designed by Frank Lloyd Wright in Florence. He sat for a long time just staring and wishing we could go inside. I wish he were alive today to see the wonderful museum and tourist attraction. Another site he liked to visit with me was Wilson Dam on the Tennessee River in Florence.

Thursday, Dec. 28, 1989

I'm at the Wilson Dam overlook. Memories. I need to go paint. It is so beautiful here. Some things never change. People still hanging out here. It is kind of nice to have a little time alone. I wish these people would leave. This place is busy. Open the flood gates!

Friday, Dec. 29, 1989

Well, it's almost time to go. Boo Hoo. I'll miss everyone very much. As usual, I want to stay longer.

Now, we're on our way. Yes, as usual, it was very difficult to say goodbye. We're in the Huntsville Jetport. I miss my mama. I'm sure it will take a little time to get over the homesickness. I want my mama. I love my mama. I love my Daddy too. I love my sister.

Mom's Journal Entries

Friday, December 29th, 1989

Boo hoo! Donnie left for L.A. Noy cooked us all breakfast. So sad for we had a wonderful week. Babe stayed off work today.

Monday, January 1, 1990

Last day of Debbie's visit. I sure hate for her to leave. Guess Babe (Babe is my Dad's nickname) was the worst. But we're going to see her and Donnie in March or April and we'll talk a lot.

Tuesday, January 2, 1990

I'm feeling a little sick at my stomach. Boo hiss and double hiss. I get so sick and tired of this damn virus. I feel it pulling at me like….…..well, like something. I'm almost in a bad mood. Definitely in a strange mood.

I guess we'll go to the market and return those movies. I would like it if God were willing for me to paint. I just need something to inspire me. I would love to paint Matthew sometimes. Maybe for practice, I should try a self-portrait.

Wednesday, January 3, 1990

It is so boring around here. What am I doing? It seems to me that I am wasting my life here. I could be out learning how to paint. I've painted for the last two nights. One was "Pot of Flowers." The other was "White Flower Against Black Background." These titles sound so artsy fartsy. So what?

As the days trickle by, I get a little more concerned about my health. Daily, I feel pulled by this virus. I'm afraid to plan and dream for the future. I ask myself daily is there any use in planning for the future. I feel drawn toward the painting. I wonder at this moment if I would have pursued my quest for art if this virus had not come along. I don't want my art to be a thing of desperation, but one of enlightenment. That sounds so corny. It is true.

Brushing Away The Tears

I'm finding a movement in my paintings. They seem, for a lack of a better word, very simple, almost like a child's painting. I guess that is where I am right now. I think the way to pursue my learning is to develop my paintings by practice. I hope this is the course I need to be on. As I said earlier, I feel time is running out.

I don't like to dwell on this aspect of my life right now. It is very depressing and sounds negative. I feel as if I'm playing a waiting game.

I'm praying for a miricle. I'm not sure if this is how one spells mirical. I was wrong. It's miracle. Thanks again Mom, for my Franklin speller!

Well the day has worn on and on. I'm at a loss as to what to do. There are many things that I would like to do with my life. Writing is possible. I never thought that I would like to write or ever enjoy it. Now I find myself writing all the time. I'm getting to the point that I would probably enjoy taking a course in journalism. One learns so much about something from doing that particular thing. Writing makes one a better writer. Painting makes one a better painter. Anyone can do anything if they display an interest in it. First comes the interest, then the ability through doing it. I do hope I become a successful artist or writer or something.

Early in 1990, Christopher and his partner began looking for a new place to live.

January 4th 1990

I painted again last night. The paintings seem to get better and better. I enjoy painting now. I feel compelled to do something every night. I can't relax until I've done something that I feel is creative.

I hope this apartment works out. I wonder if it is a good deal, considering I might not be around in the future. I guess no one really knows for sure how this thing is going to turn out. I could survive this. I hope so. I just don't want to leave Matthew with a big financial burden. He should be able to get my life insurance. God, I hope so.

** Footnote - I always knew Christopher loved me but after reading the letters he sent home, I felt the importance of his loss all over again. He was always worrying about me and the various dramas in my life. Like most little sisters with over-protective big brothers, I often felt he was interfering, so he shared his concerns with our Mom and with Matthew. I deeply miss that protective nature and unconditional love.

Letters to Mom from Christopher

Brushing Away The Tears

January 4, 1990

"I still dream about the day Matthew and I can buy our own place. I would love to own the house we live in now. We call it the yellow house (I wonder why?) Could it be that it is because like Van Gogh's house, it is yellow!

Tell Dad I need a saw. I am building my own canvases now and I definitely need a saw. I can hardly wait for you to see some of the work that I've been doing lately. I hope to have you something done by the time you get here.

January 7, 1990

I do hope Deb finds a place closer. Not only is Van Nuys inconvenient for Deb to drive every day, but I don't get to see her as much either. I'm meeting her after work, yeah!

I have to help her move a friend's sofa. And I get to get my Christmas presents from you! Mom, I say it all the time, but you are the greatest.

Deb was able to spend a little time at our house last night. It's so infrequent that we see each other. As I've said before, this will all *change once she moves in closer. We had the greatest time reading your letter. We all got a real big kick out of it.*

It was nice talking to you this morning. It is always a nice way to start out the day. I was telling Dad that Finessa (Christopher's car – He had a fun way of personifying everything) *isn't running smoothly. I think it is because I don't run her very often, and she got a little damp from the last rain.*

Had lunch with Deb and Tony. Unfortunately, she is working tonight at her part time job and has to go home first. So I guess she won't be coming over tonight. As I've said before, I just don't get to see enough of her. Is there ever enough time with those we love? Probably not.

**Footnote - After being diagnosed with AIDS, Christopher began to go to group therapy; and although it was tough at times, he knew it helped him.

Tuesday, January 9, 1990

I know it may sound a bit corny, but group was there when I needed it. I was one of those individuals who when diagnosed was misinformed if not uninformed. Group was there not only for being supportive, but it was also a wealth of information. I would have found it very difficult to deal with the whole HIV issue if group had not been there. Now that I've settled down a bit, my need has changed some. It's a good feeling to know that group will always be there. I pray and hope that I will stay healthy; and if I am in a situation where I need support, I know that group would be there.

Wednesday, January 10, 1990

I just don't feel quite useful here in this position any longer. What I need to do is sell some art. I'm not near to that point yet. I guess I'll have to wait until I see what happens. It's so hard to take, day by day. I guess I need a good old self-esteem boost. I usually get it when I'm painting something that is going well. So, I guess the remedy is to get out there and paint. Some of these people tend to make me a little intimidated. It's a problem that I've struggled with all of my life. I guess it's low self-esteem.

I think I'm experiencing a mild depression. Reading over this material, it sure sounds like it. Not a happy camper. Sometimes, I feel like I'm waiting around for someone to come up with a pill that I can take to end this nightmare. I also feel like if something doesn't happen to end this boredom I shall wig out and go berserk! Let's see, there is one more thing. Click your heels and repeat after me, ART ART ART ART ART ART ART ART ART ART.

I have many blessings to count. First on the list is Matthew. He is so important to me. He has been an absolute angel. I wonder if I would have held up as well?

**Footnote - Christopher had a strong desire to make sure his experiences with art, with AIDS, with life in general, would mean something after he was gone. His journals are peppered with references of his assumption, and fear, that no one would read what he had written. And for 12 years, no one did except his family members. I, like Christopher, feel there is much to be learned from someone's life experiences with both the living and the real possibility that the life you so love, is about to be over. Just when you think it is all doom and gloom, he ends with a quip about his spelling or some other funny aspect of life!

In the following entry, he talks about his writings and also worries that if they are read, it might make the folks he writes about mad at him.

Thursday January 11, 1990

Wow! This week has gone by extremely fast! It's almost the weekend. The days are ticking by so fast. I keep thinking I have a couple of years. Yet, I seem to be waiting to wake up one morning and have some disease or virus. Yes, that's what it feels like. Waiting to wake up and have something wrong with me. I'm sure I'm not the only one. Every time I have a spot or bump, I freak. This knowledge pushes me to the limit sometimes. I feel a strong need to produce. I think I've mentioned this before. It does keep coming up due to the circumstances. Oh well, no one may ever read this anyway. I always write this stuff because I feel that one day it might prove useful to someone somewhere. So if you are reading this now, I hope it is useful, if not sometimes amuseing. I hope this is how one spells amuseing. It's obviously not. I did look it up – AMUSING!!!!

Later...

I have another apple to sketch. Yea! Those sketches are a real challenge. Before I forget, I need to mail that letter that I just wrote for Mom.

I just thought of something that I think is funny. An apple a day keeps the doctor away. I sure hope that is true. I pray that it is true.

I just realized I'm a little hesitant to write everything. I'm afraid that people that I write about will one day read this and be upset about what I wrote. It's kind of like trying to paint a portrait of someone. *If you don't flatter them they will be very upset. I don't even want that kind of rejection down the road. That's pretty bad. I mean what are they going to do? It's not as if people will think any worse of me. If they do, so what? I don't want to be mean or anything. I just want to report what's happening in my life at this time.*

**Footnote - Christopher had a strong will. Once he decided he would do something, he focused all of his energy on that subject. Before he was diagnosed with AIDS, he would often fast. In his early stages of knowing about his disease, he also committed to fasting and eating healthier. Ironically, later he would be desperately trying to gain weight.

Wednesday, January 17, 1990

It's hump day. In more ways than one. I'm in the middle of this fast. I haven't painted at all. I really haven't felt like doing anything at all in the evening. I have these incredible headaches. I guess this fast is taking a lot out of me. I've told myself that I reserve the right to bail out at anytime. Today is supposed to be better according to the book Kurt gave me to read. I don't know. We shall see.

I'm very mellow this morning. I guess it's a result of the fast.

Monday, April 16, 1990

New Journal

Dr. Gibbs. Here I am again. A little anxious. Why? I need a therapy agenda. Sometimes it's hell to be in an OK place.

Work
Art
Relationship   W. A. R.
Where am I going???

Tuesday, April 17, 1990

Well, it's been awhile. I don't know why, but I just haven't felt compelled to write anything in these journals. Why? I think I've begun to think these things are boring. It's the same ole thing over and over. What can I say? See. What can I say is something I say all the time. What I need is more drawings and sketches and watercolors and paintings. Something of real value and not this stupid shit of pontificating all the time. Oh dear, what to draw. Draw the world, stupid. There are a million and one things to draw and I can't make up my mind sometimes. That's hard to believe, but true. What can I say?

Wednesday, April 18, 1990

One must move their day in a positive direction from the start and not wait for the day to take care of itself.

All of a sudden I found myself thinking of my Grandfather. Why, I wonder? I think it comes from reading the book on Vincent (Van Gogh).

I made a B for the mid-semester grade at school. I wanted an A. Doesn't everybody?

I'm thinking I shall continue this job and never become the artist I want to be or shall I quit and starve on the streets, but be the artist I want to be? I ask myself this and wonder is it either or.

I'm so melancholy today. I'm thinking I have lived a full life and yet I want more.

I have no reason to complain. I have experienced life in a very full way. Then why is it that I feel sorry for myself? I think I'm unwilling to embrace old age; therefore I have brought this sorrow upon myself. I just hope it is rebirth after dying or in dying. I do want to live on through my art. I've got to learn to let it go. When I do something good I need to give it away or sell it. Ha! Sell it. I wish.

Thursday April 19th, 1990

I'm here. Clinic that is. . .

As usual, I'm first. I've got to call work. I've decided to say I've had car trouble. I hate lying, but what ya gonna do? I want to say I hate this, but I won't.

Friday, April 20, 1990

Sometimes I can't make up my mind whether or not I like this job or not. Actually, I think I'm very spoiled. I don't know what I would do if I had to actually work very hard again. I was thinking about my days as a waiter and how physical that job was. I don't know. I feel like I'm passing my life away here with not very much to show for it. On the other hand, my art project is not going well. I guess that could be it. If my art is going well, then so is my life. What can I say? And that's the way it was Friday, April 20, 1990 .

On the rare days when Christopher was symptom free, he was euphoric to be alive.

Monday, April 23, 1990

Therapy tonight!!!! What's with these exclamation points? I must be a little intense. What a wonderful weekend. I felt great all weekend. My painting is going well. Very well indeed. And life is worth living, but only worth living because I'm born free.

It's raining today, and I have to drive to Dr. Gibbs. I'm so busy these days that it's very difficult to work therapy in. I wonder if I need it at times. I think I shall definitely need it in the future. It's been a saving grace these past few years, and it seems to be still working. So I should develop a better attitude. It's hi ho, hi ho, to therapy I go.

Tuesday, April 24, 1990

Yes, it's Tuesday and I survived those Monday Blues. God, they are so intense sometimes. I don't have the foggiest idea of how to deal with them either. They always, pass, usually on Tuesday; and by Wednesday I'm rolling smoothly again.

Thursday, April 26, 1990

Captain's Log

I've had such a nagging headache all day. I think it's going away for good. I've been in a melancholy mood all day. I think it had something to do with the argument we had last night. Tomorrow is Friday and I love Fridays. Yea!!! I'm excited already. Class tonight. I hope to get a lot done. I've really got to get down and start the details on my painting. First I must re-do the color of my colander.

I never seem to really get down and enter things in this ledger of real deep down meaning. Why? I'm afraid someone might read it.

I'm not feeling that well today. I feel like I need a long break, a nice long rest. One of those days where I could sleep in for a long time. I didn't get to do that this past weekend. Maybe next weekend I shall.

Later: I'm feeling better. Thank God! I think I shall go to the party the firm is having tonight. Actually I had rather go home and paint. That is what I would really like to do.

On other fronts:

Well, my painting. I think I'm going to like my painting very much. The colors are wonderful. I hope to get at least an A-, well maybe a B. I think the problem here is that it doesn't fit the criteria of a classical still life.

Monday, April 30, 1990

Facing the Monday Blues again. I must get out of here before my mind snaps and nothing will ever be the same. I think a good book would do the trick. Actually, doing these journals helps. I do need to practice my typing. I rarely, if ever, type for real anymore. I wonder if you could call this for real? I know that it is pretty bad. At this point I shall ask you, the reader, how am I doing? Am I boring you to tears? Do you think I'm stupid because for all the typos? I could go on and on and on and on and on and on. Do you know how difficult it is go keep repeating something on the typewriter? Very! I think I've written enough for now. So long Toots, and adieu and chow and all that stuff. Oh yes, I almost forgot Adieus Amigos.

Tuesday, May 1, 1990

Thank God the Monday Blues are out of the way. Now, maybe I can jump into the week. It's now mid-afternoon and the day has moved along smoothly. I have not felt that well yesterday or today. Why? Why do you think? I have this damn nagging stomach problem. I need to get off the coffee. Ok, Christopher, stop it now!!!!! From this moment I shan't have a cup of coffee until the next one. If it's not one thing, it's another. Life sometimes is a bitch, and it goes on an on on an on. I just wish I felt better. I shall. This usually passes as time goes on.

I need to paint tonight. God, let me paint tonight. Matthew got his job today. Yea! He really is going to take off. Me, well I'm kind of stuck here. I guess it could be worse. I mean this isn't so bad. It does allow time for things like journal entries. I just hope my art blossoms and continue to grow. I do wish it would grow faster. This means I need to spend more time on it, which I find hard to do with this job. I need more time to devote to my art. ART ART ART ART ART ART ARTARTARTARTARTARTARTARTART!!!!

Tuesday, May 8, 1990

The car is out again. What's new about that? I've decided on what painting I shall use for my Masterpiece project. Naturally it's a Van Gogh. Starry Night. The day is rather dragging. I live in fear of starting to feel badly. I felt great this morning and now, well I don't really feel that great. I need some purpose in my life. I sit here, day after day, and feel nothing but despair over feeling I'm wasting away here. It's the same old song over and over. I've had these same feelings before. What I need to do is some good work. So get out there and paint, paint.

Tuesday, May 15, 1990

I painted last night and it went fairly well. I'm beginning to believe in myself as a painter again. I'm a little concerned about the time

I'm able to devote to the craft. I'm ready to take off again and zoom. I hope this isn't a false feeling. I haven't learned to trust my belief in myself, that I'm special and that I have something special to say.

I haven't been drawing at all lately. I think it's because I haven't been feeling that well physically. The other reason could be that I'm just not disciplined enough. I was doing so well there for a while. The creative tide ebbs and flows, ebbs and flows.

**Footnote - In the following entry, what starts out as somewhat typical, ends as one of the most heartbreaking of all the journal entries. It has stayed in my mind and heart and the ending to the entry echoes in my head often – "It's so difficult sometimes. I don't want them to hurt. I do want them to miss me." I guess that is the way many terminal patients feel. What Christopher didn't realize is that you can't miss someone and not hurt. The two emotions go together. I remember thinking in the first few hours after he died that at least he would never have to suffer the intense pain of losing a parent or a sibling.

He also spoke in this entry of having the easy part – "All I have to do is die. I think that may be the simple part."

Wednesday, May 16, 1990

Brushing Away The Tears

Today Matthew and I discussed my advancement options at the law firm. I need to give this some thought. I feel pretty stuck to tell the truth. This could just be a part of my ambivalence toward things as of late. I just don't know what has gotten into me. I think it could be the fact that I have clinic tomorrow. I always seem to get like this before my appointment. It's always the same. So get over it, girl. Matthew if you ever read this, go ahead and laugh. Yes, I'm getting morbid.

My painting went well last night. I have a lot to do as far as that class is concerned.

I seem to be at odds today with the people I work with. Not really into disagreements or anything, just not in harmony. Again, it could be the fact that I have clinic tomorrow. No matter what I try and write about it starts to sound depressing. Again clinic. I'm beginning to think I don't like clinic. I just don't want to get sick yet. I have so much to do. Every time I feel this way I think I'm getting sick, and the end is near. I know Matthew feels that way also, and I don't know how to deal with that. I know we've talked about it before, but we need to deal with it. I don't want to fool myself into believing that I'm going to lick this thing. It is possible, but maybe not; and we should be prepared to face that. It's so painful not just for me, but him. All I have to do is die. I think that may be simple part. I know it will be more difficult on them than me.

Handwritten – It's so difficult sometimes… I don't want them to hurt…

I do want them to miss me.

Friday May 18, 1990

I have to work tomorrow. I have a slight feeling that my meningitis is coming back. Maybe not, but I keep getting those feelings. I hope not. It could be that I'm just getting paranoid. We shall see.

My painting went well last night. Thank God!! I must paint this weekend. I pray that the paint moves. We shall see. I can never tell whether or not the paints will move or not. So far it is hit and miss.

Our trip comes up this week!!! I can hardly wait. I know that Matthew is really looking forward to it. I love him so much. He's like a little kid sometimes. I know he doesn't believe it, but he is so innocent sometimes.

Wednesday May 23, 1990

Yes!!! Yes!!! Yes!!! It's almost here. Vacation that is. Tomorrow is the day. Amsterdam here we come. I'm in such a good mood today. I wonder why? Could it be called vacation? Anyway, the day is moving along so well.

My painting went fantastic last night. I think I may be onto something.

Matthew sent flowers today. I'm telling you life just doesn't get much better. I do want to keep improving as an artist. This is my goal as of now.

**Footnote - Christopher and Matthew traveled to Amsterdam on vacation in late May of 1990. He was filled with wonder at the art he had traveled so far to see, a Van Gogh exhibit.

Monday, June 4, 1990

I'm back. Back from Europe that is. What a trip. I just can't believe that it's over. The art. My God! The art!!!!! I hope I can hold onto that feeling. You know that feeling of Europe. The only problem now is that I feel stifled as an artist. This city is ugly now and so smoggy. What am I going to do? I'll just have to find things to paint. First, I'll have to learn to paint. Ah ha that sounds good to me.

After seeing all the art of Van Gough, it kind of makes me ashamed of my output. Will I ever be able to do that kind of work or at least that amount? Again and again I ask myself, am I ready to embark on my career as an artist? I think this will take total commitment. Am I ready to give up my job security? I think there will come a time to really seriously consider these questions, but for now I have got to get in there and learn how to be the best damn artist that I can.

The quest has begun. I began it when I took that first drawing class in 1988. Now, I'm up to painting and moving along. I must! And I repeat I must learn as much as fast as I can. It's imperative! Even under the best of circumstances I am behind, and the circumstances aren't that great as it is.

Wednesday, June 6, 1990

I'm definitely bored again. I don't know – things seem to be moving along, yet they seem to have no definite importance. I want importance attached to my daily doings. I think that is what I'm seeking in my art. Something of importance. I really don't think anyone here values me or the work I do. I mean it's so menial. I go through each day and feel like I am just biding my time. I know in the long haul it is paying off. I want reward now, at this very moment. I need instant gratification. I want recognition. I want acceptance. Now, Now, Now, Now, Now, Now, Now!

Tuesday, June 5, 1990

There is this new guy in the office and he is sort of a queen. Actually, he is a queen. I feel that he is another misfit and we will probably become friends. That is the way it usually goes. I pair up with the strangest characters.

Wednesday, June 6, 1990

Day three back at work. The glow of vacation is definitely wearing off. This place reeks of insincerity. "How are you? Fine. And how are you?" To hear it in person is quite disgusting. I'm obviously not in a very good mood this morning. Why? It could be a lot of things.

Monday, June 11, 1990

I know I should consider myself lucky in that I have the time to devote to these journals. I mean I get to write in them daily. I think it is predestined that I should do so. After all it is for prosperity that I'm doing it in the first place. Remember me.

Wednesday, June 13, 1990

Every time I have Clinic I get so stressed out about it the day before that it makes me depressed or crazy or both. I must say that I am always on a high afterwards, though. Get it over with and get on with other more important things. I should really acknowledge the importance of Clinic and put it in its proper perspective. It is important!

Tomorrow keeps coming up. I always get the feeling that I'm inconveniencing Mathew. It's probably just me, but it feels that way sometimes. What can I say. I think I get in these funks every time before Clinic.

Thursday, June 14, 1990

It's over. Clinic that is! I'm so happy I can't even tell you. It's not that bad, it's just the whole ordeal. Driving down there and back, waiting in the lines, seeing all those sick people. The positive side of that is that I really get treated very well by all of the staff. It's amazing how well I get treated there. I think those people like me.

On the subject of art. I feel I must get on the ball. I have a destiny to fulfill. I need to draw and draw in order to be able to paint. My final goal is painting. Well, actually I think I might be interested in sculpter down the road. I think I should learn to spell it first. S C U L P T U R E. That's it, sculpture. Really Christopher, sometimes I think you have the inclinations of being stupid. I think I need to read my Van Gogh books.

"Sometimes it seems like I'm never going to get home again. It's so far and out of sight," I don't know why I included this. It's a passage from a song back in the 60's. Actually, it's "gonna make it home again and not get home again."

I yelled at Matthew last night. I hate it when I do that. I don't know what makes me fly off the handle like that. The odd thing is that I was talking about anger in my therapy session last night. Now why would I lash out at Matthew? I need to watch it though. He is truly good to me, and I should treat him better. It don't matter who was right or wrong. When one yells like that the battle is over, and it doesn't matter if you are right or wrong, you lose.

Christopher did not share with his co-workers that he was sick with AIDS. His insurance with the firm had a three year pre-existing rule. Also, like thousands of other HIV and AIDS sufferers, he didn't know how they would react and could not bear to be talked about and seen as an outcast, *even in Los Angeles*. Because of this giant secret, he had to lie about his clinic appointments. This was very difficult for him. Honesty was important to Christopher, in himself, and in others.

Tuesday, June 1990 (look up date)

Well, Monday is out of the way. One would think I didn't like my job or life from a statement like that. In some ways that is true. There are aspects of my life that I am having a difficult time at the moment. I hate to juggle my time around. I'll be more specific. I hate to lie once a month about why I have to be out ½ day. I was told today that when I make up time I must be able to prove that I did have something to do. It's bad enough that I have to go to that damn appointment, but to have to make up the time and then have to justify the time. Boo hiss. Woe is me. Poor little ole me, and so on and so on.

I must find my way. I am experiencing periods of total confusion. The only thing that seems to anchor me is my drawing. I feel the need to draw to rescue me. At this very moment I am drifting. I need out! I need something to bring me to shore.

How at this point can I call myself an Artist? I am at the beginning and still have a lot to learn. I do have the drive and desire, but will that see me through? I have a feeling that I will be successful, but can I bide my time until that happens? This is the question. Not whether I will achieve my goals, but can I stand the wait?

I feel like I'm in Artist Hell at the moment. This waiting for the moment when I shall be able to create and do, not sit here and wait for the moment. Shall I survive? This is a good question. A question that I hope has a happy ending. Time keeps dragging on and on and on. One can only hope that he reaches his potential in his lifetime. If we only had a way of knowing this. It's the waiting that gets unbearable and the not knowing, especially the not knowing.

Monday July 2, 1990

I had a strange weekend. I was sick for most of it. I thought this is it. Actually, I knew it wasn't it. I thought it could have been food poisoning. Come to find out it was the flu. It has been going around in our office. The tragic thing is that I didn't do any art at all weekend. That really is sickening. I didn't go to the gym yesterday either. I was just too sick. I can't believe it, but actually considered it all day. I think it has become an obsession. Not necessarily the actual workout, but the way it makes me feel and look! I am amazed sometimes in the progress I'm making on this front.

Tuesday, July 3, 1990

I'm sick. Yes, I have a flu that is going around and I feel lousy.

4:35, and will soon be time to go home. I am feeling much better. I was a little worried there for a while, especially last night. I really did feel rotten. I think I'm on the way to recovery. Let's hope so.

**Footnote - The 4th of July was special that year as my brother spent it with me. Also, as his office was close to mine at the Bonaventure Hotel, I started to spend many lunch hours with him and those times were always memorable.

THE POSITIVE THINKING PERIOD

Many of his writings would have a fatalistic tone or reference, despite his attempts to stop pessimistic musings. To counter the pessimism, he started to engage in daily positive thinking meditations.

Thursday, July 4, 1990

The fourth is over and now there is the weekend to look forward to. I can hardly wait.

Yesterday was great. I did a sketch of a dead orchid plant at Deb's house. It turned out very nice. I think I should have a few of my things matted.

Deb's bringing lunch today. Great! I can hardly wait.

It's much later and will soon be 3:00 . Break time. I can hardly wait. I hope to do a study.

I've actually had another small bout with this damn flu. A small case of diarrhea. I think I'm going to be OK. It's just that it makes me feel so bad. So bad that I don't feel like drawing and that is bad.

Friday, July 6, 1990

Today is Friday and it started off weird. I just can't seem to get it together. For one reason or another. I woke up sick to my stomach and sweating.

Deb is coming for lunch. I can hardly wait!

It will soon be time for all of us to make major decisions. Like what you ask? What will we want, and where will we be?

I'm just thinking if anybody reads this they will think I'm definitely off my rocker. Speaking of rockers. No, I won't say anything. It's time to get started on my life. What's left of it. Christopher stop it right now. This is really a strange day. Can't you tell?

Monday, July 6, 1990

I'm now at peace with the universe. I know it sounds corny, but hey if it works then it works. I've started going through this exercise where I reaffirm my existence and well being. For example, I am at peace with the universe, I feel energy flowing through and around me, I'm a creative being, everything has its place and I have mine. This gives you some idea of what I'm talking about. I hope I can develop this and take it to its limits.

It's almost 4:00 and I have had a very good day. I managed several good studies. I think the reason I'm so into drawing today is that I got some new pencils yesterday and they have set my ass on fire.

Tuesday, July 10, 1990

I'm trying to keep up my positive attitude today. I know it sounds stupid, but hey I'll try anything.

I feel positive that good things will come my way today. I will embrace them and take them and use them to my advantage. I feel energy about me around me and moving through me. I will look at other people in a more positive forging light. Light shall come into my life and surround me protecting me from all negative energy.

I wish they would find a cure for this damn thing. I say this because I don't dare utter the word in this place. I feel like I'm in prison sometimes. Christopher, stop it. Start your positive thinking.

** Footnote - As I mentioned earlier, Christopher was in constant fear that his co-workers would find out about his illness.

Wednesday, July 11, 1990

Well, it is now about 3:40, and it will soon be time to go home. I should say time to go Dr. Gibbs. I wonder what I'll talk about tonight? Sometimes it seems like I have nothing on the ole agenda. At times, I think I should drop therapy, then again under the circumstances, I think not. Those circumstances we all know, but I don't dare disclose here for fear of exposure. What a life.

Think positive. I am at peace with the world. I am in harmony with the world. I feel energy moving around me and about me. I shall have a positive attitude about people around me and whom I come in contact with.

I did a couple of studies today. Nothing that was earth shattering or anything. The thing is that I must draw, and draw and draw if I am to reach my goals. My goals are that of becoming a fantastic artist. Art on Christopher.

List for Clinic

Flu
Memory Loss
Hair Loss

Thursday, July 12, 1990

I did Clinic again. As usual it wasn't so bad. As usual I always dread it more than I should. It was nice having Matthew along with me. It made the trip much better.

I didn't do any art last night. For one reason or the other. I did have Dr. Gibbs, and I was late for that. I couldn't remember if the appointment was a 6:00 or 7:00, it was neither – it was 6:30. So I missed almost thirty minutes of my appointment. I asked my practitioner about the memory thing, and she said that they have noted that there has been some memory loss.

During the summer of 1990 Christopher had a period of relatively good health. It would be the last good summer for him. He used it to focus on maintaining a positive attitude and on enjoying his life.

July 13, 1990

I did a couple of studies today. One I'm calling, "the party is over." It's a study of some balloons that have been around for quite some time and partially deflated.

I go home next week. 4 days only, but it should be very interesting. I hope to do some drawings while there. This should prove to be profitable, hopefully. Profitable in that it gives me an opportunity to do some drawings of the country.

July 16, 1990

Yes, it's good ole Monday again. Interesting day though. It seems like it has fun smoothly. I have been able to avoid the Monday Blues for two Mondays in a row. Lucky me.

I had my first summer painting class yesterday. Boring! I think I can make it work out, but it was sort of a waste of time yesterday. Think positive. This reminds me that I haven't done my positive thinking exercises as of today so here goes.

I am at peace with the world. I am in harmony with the universe. I am in harmony with the people around me and the things about me. I am tranquil. I feel positive energy moving around me and through me. I am at peace. I can visualize a hill with rain falling down gently and daisies all around me. I am at peace and the world is a nice place to be and I am OK and things are as they should be. I at peace. PEACE.

I'm writing Greta a letter. I think some of it sounds sort of corny. I do think in some ways she is one of the only people who probably really, I mean really, understands me. I think we come from the same place in many respects. I think she has that same creative streak that unless she satisfies it then she will always be restless. She is one of the only people, other than Matthew, that I can look to for guidance. With Matthew its one kind of guidance and with her it's a totally different type. I need creative input and she is one of the only people I know that I can look to for it.

July 17, 1990

Today is my Friday! It feels like it too. I think this is going to be an absolutely wonderful day. I've got a lot to do to prepare for this trip.

Some people are so homophobic. I mean really. The sad thing about that is that I find it sort of attractive. I think it has to do with the fact that they are unavailable.

**Footnote - It has always been interesting to me that people who have good relationships with their parents and family, refer to going "home." Such was the case with Christopher.

Wednesday, July 18, 1990

6:20 , LAX terminal, Southwest Gate 7, #1 & #2 boarding passes. Alabama , here we come!!!

Monday July 23, 1990

I'm back. Back from Alabama that is. It's truly like a dream. I can't believe it's all over. I truly would of liked to have stayed awhile longer. Maybe a month or so. I must think positive and if it is meant to be, then it will happen.

JOURNAL ENTRY FROM MOM

Monday, July 23, 1990

Got my painting today from Donnie, UPS. Finally got my anniversary gift from Donnie. It is beautiful. Donnie did it in art school, a Van Gogh. He made an A on it. I'm so glad he loves me enough to give it to me.

Christopher adored our niece Katy. He especially wanted her to visit Los Angeles. The two of us bought her plane tickets for her high school graduation present during the summer of 1990.

July 27, 1990

It's that day again. Thank God!!! This weekend should prove to be a good one. Katy's here, and we should so some interesting things. I am looking forward to them.

I need to do my positive thing exercises.

I am at peace with the world and universe. I am in harmony with myself and the world around me. I am tranquil and calm. I am in a positive mood. Positive energy is moving through me and around me. I am at peace. I am in a positive mood. I am at peace.

July 31, 1990

I need more responsibility around the office. I need to start looking for ways to make myself more useful. We shall see. I must learn to trust in the fates. I feel I am being guided along some inner path. I think it is going to bart, then again life can be strange.

I need to do some correspondence. Greta, Lola and Mom, of course.

Brushing Away The Tears

August 1, 1990

This day has turned out to be quite nice. Very positive indeed. I managed to do a couple of pastel studies. One of an Iris turned out very nice. A 15 minute break is just not enough time to do a masterpiece. I shall keep at it though.

** - Footnote He often did positive-thinking exercises for Matthew and me.

August 6, 1990

I feel positive energy moving around me and through me. I am happy and content. Now for my sister. I feel that my sister will be at peace with herself and the world around her. I feel good things are going to happen to her today. I feel positive energy moving through around and through her. She is happy and content. She is successful and will have the job she deserves.

I think I shall start a new journal here and call it the Yellow House. STUDIO STUDIO STUDIO STUDIO STUDIO STUDIO!!!!

THE YELLOW HOUSE PERIOD

August 7, 1990

New journal! A new beginning. I feel great and the future looks bright. I shall soar today and everyday here after.

I have some new art materials. Curtis gave me a set of markers, colored pencils, regular drawing pencils and charcoals. A new medium. I haven't even learned pastels as of yet and now something new.

This day is coming to a close. The work day that is. I did three studies, not very good, but still I did them. I do hope that I learned something from them, this is my hope. I shall continue to grow and grow as an Artist. This is the dream, and this is the hope.

Wednesday, August 8, 1990

I'm going to start this out by doing some positive thinking exercises for my sister.

Debbie will be happy. She will have a very positive day and positive things will come her way. All negativity will pass away and she will obtain the goals and things in her life that she needs.

Now for Matthew. Matthew is happy and content. Good things will happen to him today. Positive energy is moving around him and through him. Good things will happen to him today.

I'm having a fantastic day. I've been creative. I did another study during break today. It was an interesting situation of study in perspective and I don't think I got it exactly right.

I have clinic tomorrow. Oh well, it could be worse. At least I have the whole day off. I also have to register for class. I guess I should say classes. I still want to go to Otis and maybe it will still work out.

August 28, 1990

Wow! What a weekend! We got so much accomplished. We're in the Yellow House. I can hardly believe it. It's like a dream come true. It is a dream come true. Now if I can only get in there and start painting. This has been a goal all along. So I need to get in there and do it!

I hate feeling this way. It could be worse. I mean this constant nagging stomach ache. I also keep trying to get this nagging headache, accompanied by a stomach ache. What can I do? Suffer!

August 30, 1990

Mom and Dad arrive tonight. Yea, I am really excited and looking forward to them seeing our new house. The Yellow House. We have a lot to do. The studio is coming along great. I finally got the shelves up and the place straightened up. Looks great. Now for some art. It seems like I don't really have the time with all the things we have to do with getting the house ready. I do love that house and I guess I'll have to make allowances. I do hope to do some fab art there.

September 6, 1990

At Dr. Gibbs. I'm so afraid of writing what I really feel anymore. Why? I wonder if I know what I feel anymore. It feels as if I. . . I'm adrift. Tossed around and about. I don't know what I want. I'm not unhappy...yet, I seem to be missing something. What?

**Footnote - Christopher often wrote our mother long, detailed letters about his art projects.

Letter from Christopher to Mom January 14, 1991

Dear Mom,

I'm still working on my landscape series. It's funny, but I couldn't for the life of me decide what I wanted to do tonight in class and while writing this to you I figured it out.

I turned in my self-portrait last night. I thought I could make a C at the most.

Letter from Christopher to Mom, January 21, 1991

Mom, I made A's in my final art projects last night! I'm really basking in the afterglow of it all. It's so nice to finally be good in something. I mean really good. My teacher thinks this series of paintings is salable. I value her opinion in that she also teaches at Otis Parsons, which is one of the best art schools on the West Coast. I took classes there a few times. I'm so excited about the prospects of finally being able to do something that I enjoy and making a go of it somewhere down the road.

I know I've told you this before, but I have it on my mind these days. I thought it might be like a lot of other paths I've gone down in my life and not come to anything, but so far this has not been the case. It's seems that I'm heading down a path and though I'm having to find my way, I'm not growing neither weary nor tired of it. I know this sounds a bit poetic, but I have a romantic attachment to my art.

New Journal. This will be a great journal.

Monday, February 11, 1991

Got Deb's painting under way. It's going well. Needs quite a bit of refining, but that will come.

** Footnote - The painting depicted a beautiful vase of flowers for Valentine's Day. He told me that the flowers were forever and would never wilt or die. He wrote on the back on the canvas, "To the best sister in the world. I love you very much."

Monday is almost out of the way. It's terrible to have this attitude about time. Time should not be wasted; it should be appreciated. I need to keep this in mind and stop wishing my time away. I must learn that I'm where I need to be and lucky to be there. I need to make use of every moment. I need to stop worrying about what's next and learn to live and love every moment of every day. This sounds corny, but there is a lot of truth in it. Practice this in positive thinking exercises.

Monday, February 25, 1991

I've got to find a way out of here. I'm hoping that my art will lead the way out. Will it? I know this is not the function of art, but it seems to be my only hope.

How does one rule out negativity? Good question. I miss you Dr. Gibbs. I'm so full of negativity. I wonder why. It's a wonder I'm not out mowing people down. I have so much anger that it frightens me.

It's time to call it a day and get ready for the evening. Adieu to you and you and you and you and you and you………

Friday, March 1, 1991

I'm feeling a bit trapped here again. Why? I'm not making enough money, that's why. What to do? Sell some paintings, that's what. I must get in there and do a large enough body of work that I will improve to the point that I can produce something that the public will have to have. This means work, work, work.

Wednesday, March 27, 1991

I have a new small canvas that I'm going to do a painting of some lilies. This painting is going to be for my aunt Bobby Sue. I guess this is good practice for those upcoming commissions. I think this is hoping, but I think my painting is getting ready to take a new and fast turn. I hope so.

I'm continuing my studies of Matisse. What a painter. He gives me both hope and despair. I say this because he still mystifies me in a way.

** Footnote - The ugly head of AIDS-related illnesses began to rear its ugly head again in April of 1991.

Monday, April 1, 1991

Am I getting sick? This is the question on my mind at the moment. I just can't seem to shake this flu bug.

Tuesday, April 2, 1991

The painting went well this morning. So much so that I think I'm planning to drop my class at PCC. This of for one reason or another mostly because of the time factor.

I'm still a little under the weather. I feel much better than yesterday and am having hopes of full recovery this time. It really scares me in the worst way when something like this lingers.

I need to call Dr. Gibbs. I need to go in for a consultation, or what you might call a tune up.

Wednesday, April 3, 1991

Well, it seems that I'm over this flu. I was really worried there for a while. This flu thing really put a dent in my physical well being. Not only did it affect me physically, it put a dent in my emotional self as well. I still feel a little weak from it all and will for a while. This has made me seriously consider going off sugar, milk and hopefully, eventually coffee. I've got to get my physical self back together. Will this nightmare ever end?

I called Dr. Gibbs today. I left a message that I wanted to schedule a session with him. Yes, it has come to this. I need to work some things out. We shall see what he says.

Monday, April 8, 1991

Am I sick? This so called flu keeps coming back. I can't seem to shake it completely. One day I'm fine, the next I feel like crap. I'm terribly frightened. Is this the beginning of the end? This is the big question. I don't think so, but maybe I'm being optimistic. When will this nightmare end? It has to at some point. I must say that I should get things in order though. I need to go back in and organize these journals. Enough of this doom and gloom, because at the moment I feel great, well, maybe not great; but I feel pretty good.

These journals have become more or less a novel. It seems like I'm writing these entries to someone else and not to me. A book of my life. Documentation. Is this what I want? Is this fulfilling any needs? I can see them serving some uses, but to what avail? Questions, questions. I need answers.

Tuesday, April 9, 1991

My strength is going, or so it feels. I must do something about it. I feel fine in all other areas. I've got to get to the bottom of this. It feels as though I'm operating on a low battery. I do see the doctor Thursday. Maybe this will help. At the moment I wish I could just go home and sleep for a long time. This is impossible so I'll struggle through the day. I feel that I'm trying to do all the right things such as eating right. Enough of this. I don't think I need to say anymore except that I'm worried.

Thursday, April 11, 1991

We found the cat. Dead. What a nightmare. It was from the fumigating in the house. There is so much sadness in the world. This is only the tip of the iceberg. I'm still not up to 100% of my health level. I doubt if I'll ever be. This cat thing is just one more sad thing to add to the list that seems to be growing weekly.

I do have good things in my life at the moment such as Matthew and my painting. The painting is coming along nicely.

I have Dr. Gibbs tonight. First time in a long time. Is this admission of failure? I don't think so. I'm definitely stuck at the moment. I need to move through this and into something new. I can't say I'm bored. I think I'm just tired. Physically tired.

It seems like I'm back in the same old position. That of wondering what my purpose is here. I was so busy here at work for a while, now nothing. I question my own existence. I think the problem is that I'm severely depressed. The cat thing has really upset me to the utmost. I know it sounds corny, but time heals all wounds or at least makes them bearable.

I'm feeling so washed out. Will I ever have a bloom on my cheeks again? I hope so. I'm trying to do everything that I can to make it happen. If it does I'll be so happy. I need some energy. It's so difficult to explain. I feel fine, it's just my energy is so low. I feel like I'm in a haze or fog. It is true that I've been having only one cup of coffee compared to my usual 4 or 5 a day. I've cut down on my sugar to almost the point that I don't have any. These things could be factors in my energy level, but I seem to panic and live in fear that it's the start of the end. I guess though in reality the end starts the day we're born.

I so hope this week will be a week of painting. This is why I want to go home (to Alabama). I shall try my best to make it a painting trip.

I think I'll be glad I did when I return and have a painting or two to show for my week's efforts.

Friday, April 12, 1991

Day before blast off! Am I ready? More ready today than yesterday. I feel so much better today. I think I'm really over this bout of being ill.

Tuesday, April 23, 1991

Back from Alabama. I'm over this intestinal thing, and now I'm having a back problem. Will it ever end?

I did two paintings in AL. One of Mom's Irises and one of Dad's shop.

I'm a bit concerned about this back problem. It seems like it's one thing after another.

I wish we didn't have to worry about finances. I would love to be able to go home for a couple of months and paint till I couldn't paint no more.

Wednesday, April 24, 1991

I'm feeling much better today. I think this back thing must be resolving itself. I certainly hope so. I do wish my health problems would improve. It's been hell these few months. I need to feel better in order to paint better. The beat goes on.

Thursday, April 25, 1991

Busy again here at work. This is good in that I don't have time to sit around and wonder about my existence.

My hair is falling out by handfuls. I think some of it could be the medication and some of it could be age. It's so difficult to tell these days. My health has been on the blink more or less this whole year. I just don't feel very good anymore. Sometimes I feel ok for a brief time, but it's usually very brief.

Friday, April 26, 1991

I'm reworking another painting. The small white studio landscape. I'm really enjoying this, but I feel I need to be moving on to something else. Reworking these paintings made me realize how much I've grown as a painter since the original execution of these works.

**Footnote – Ironically, our Dad once was a painter, of a different sort – commercial and industrial while my brother was an artistic kind of painter.

I'm still trying to absorb Matisse. I feel a bit frustrated in that it's so obvious that he has a lot of art education. How much can a person learn on his own? Good question. I have one thing on my mind at the moment. MATISSE. It's what carries me through these boring days. Is he my hope and salvation? I use to think Van Gogh was, and I'll always be indebted to him and he was my first love. I think I may even have an attraction for Picasso. Imagine that.

** Footnote - A few nights after Christopher died, I looked up at the stars and thought, perhaps now Christopher can paint with the masters and extract the knowledge from them that he was so eager to learn.

Wednesday, May 22, 1991

Clinic tomorrow. It's been 8 weeks since I've been to the doctor and I think it's about time I went.

Monday June 3, 1991

I feel that I'm advancing with my art at a snail's pace. 20 – 30 minutes a day with a few hours on the weekend doesn't make it. Is there any hope of attaining the goals that I want to attain in the time that I have?

Friday June 7, 1991

I've made it through another week. It's had its ups and downs; mostly ups, and I guess that is what counts. My health is better, and I think the intestinal thing may be cleared up. I hope so in that it was really a pain to say the least and had me very worried.

LOSING HIS LOOKS

As the summer of 1991 progressed, Christopher became increasingly worried about his appearance.

Monday, June 10, 1991

I'm in a semi-depressed state. I'm very depressed about losing my hair. It is really falling out now. I don't know how much of it from stress and how much of it is from the drugs. I don't feel that attractive anymore. The bloom is definitely gone. I don't think there is any getting it back either. I'm sick of the gym and I'm sick of being sick. I'm sick, sick! I guess you could say that I'm really depressed.

The more things I accomplish in my life, the more I want. A year ago I would have been ecstatic to have accomplished the things that I have in the past year. Now, it's not enough. I want more. Looking back at the paintings I've done...they're not good enough. This frustrates me a lot. They're good enough for me, but I want them to be really good. Good enough to hang on other peoples walls. I want to sell them. I know this is so shallow, but in the light of my current job, it's almost absolutely necessary. This brings me back around to the financial thing that is depressing me in the first place.

Tuesday, June 11, 1991

I have diarrhea again this morning. It's the second morning in a row that I'm getting a little concerned and I think I should mention it to my Dr.

Lunch is over and I'm still not feeling all that well. I don't know what this is, but I do wish it would go away. I think if it doesn't it will wear me out. I'm already feeling a bit down from it. It seems like this nightmare will never end. Maybe in death, but I don't want to talk about that now. I think this will pass, as everything else has;

but it sure is inconvenient. I want a new body. I might not ought to wish for this in that I might just get my wish. Enough of this!

Tuesday, June 18, 1991

Well, clinic is out of the way. Thank God! I don't have to go back for 4 weeks. This was fantastic news. I do hope they come up with something and soon. I don't know how long I can go on like this in that it really gets to me sometimes.

I was finally able to pull that acrylic together. It was a tough job, but I managed. It seems I pour a lot of my life into those paintings. I spend so much time with them that they become a part of me. This is the reason I have such a difficult time giving them up as a failure.

Letter to Mom from Christopher

Wednesday June 19, 1991

Dear Mom,

I can't believe it but this is the first time I've even attempted to write this week. Why? I think I've been more or less depressed here lately. I think it could be because of clinic this week. I don't know why, but I'm terribly depressed during those weeks that I have to go and now I have to go every 4 weeks. I'm sure it will pass. I think part of it could be because of the fact that my painting is in a transition period.

I think I told you that I'm now working with a new type of paints. They're called Acrylics and they're a water based paint and so much easier to work with. I just haven't quite got the hang of them yet. I have done one nice painting with them and I really liked the way they worked, but this second painting isn't going as well so I think it brings me down a bit.

Work has been rather hectic at times. Some days I'm so busy here that I can't catch my breath and then others, just nothing. On those days that I don't do much I start to question my existence. At times I do wonder why and what am I doing here at this job. At one time I would have been happy in this position, but now it's not enough and I feel a little trapped. So the story goes. I'll pass through this, I always do. I'm really tired though. I know you know what I mean in that I think we all feel this way at times. I'm lucky in that I don't get this way very often, but when I do it's a doosey. What I need is some of your TLC and home cooking. It seems that I just can't seem to get out of this complaining mode so I'll close until Friday when Ill finish this up. Adieu.

Friday

It's Friday and clinic is out of the way. For a long time. This is the longest I've ever had to go between visits. This is fantastic news in that we all know how much I love going. It was so nice hearing that I'm in great health. I'm still a little concerned about this intestinal flu bug. Still seem to have a touch of it.

Love to all of you and I'll be seeing everyone soon.

Christopher

Wednesday, June 26, 1991

This workday is coming to a close. I don't know what it is but I've been in a rather strange place here today. I think I need some rest. I feel rather burned out. I look in the mirror and I don't like what I see anymore. I look old. Have I aged that much in the past couple of years? Looking at what I've gone through it's no wonder. I just wish I could tell what is natural aging and what is from being sick. I seem to do all the right things, such as getting enough of sleep, not drinking very much alcohol, using skin conditioner and hair products. I do all of the above and I still look beat and tired. Will I ever have a bloom in my cheek? It's rather depressing. Am I just ugly? I wouldn't say ugly, but barely passable. I would like to at least feel a little energetic. I guess my reserves are low. My artistic capabilities are rather high at the moment, and I guess that is something.

Friday, July 5, 1991

Back at work. Boo!

I think the Dapsone is making me sick again. I discontinued it this morning and plan to take it up again on Monday. I hope that I eventually can tolerate it. I don't want to be going to clinic every 4 weeks. I do wish they would come up with something that would end this nightmare. There is so much that I want from life at the moment. There is so much that I want to do and get done. Not only in art, but things I want to see and places that I want to revisit. Will I get to do these things? I shall try.

A letter from me to Mom, February 27, 1992

Dear Homefolks,

We are going to leave a few minutes early today because I have therapy at 6 and last week I was late because of traffic. Christopher is supposed to treat me to lunch at Taipan, A Chinese restaurant in his building. I hope he can eat and enjoy it.

We are so busy today, not a good day to leave early. But Sherry (my boss) says it's OK. Also tomorrow I have to drive Christopher to Torrance to pick up the sample bottles and leave a sample if he can. Can you believe his doctor forgot to leave them so he could pick them up Saturday?

It was nice to stay home this weekend. I napped and read yesterday and watched a little TV (which I rarely have time to do these days). Also, I'm hooked on the Gameboy Nintendo game! My therapist says that is good for me because it does totally absorb you! The only game I play right now is the Super Mario Brothers. It's like the big game Katy and Donnie play so much.

Time to get this in the mail. Take care and I miss and love you all.

Love, Debbie

**Footnote - In April of 1992, Mom and Dad visited me and Christopher for more than a week. Christopher wanted Dad to come in the spring to help him plant some tomatoes and a few other vegetable garden items. (I took pictures of Dad and Christopher planting the garden).

Excerpts from Mom's journal of the Los Angeles trip.

Tuesday April 21, 1992

Got up early, lots to do. Deb and Christopher met us at the airport with signs saying, "Hazel and Babe". It was such a glorious moment, to be hugging and kissing them again. I savored the moment. We came to Deb's home in Burbank . Matthew came and picked Christopher up as he was getting tired.

Friday April 24, 1992

A beautiful day. I'm not cooking tonight, pot luck. We went driving and shopping and Babe bought Christopher a pair of suspenders at K mart. He came home with Deb and we heated up supper, and then watched TV. Christopher lay down for a while.

Saturday April 25, 1992

Las Vegas! Got up early. Donnie called and said he feels great and is going with us! Wonderful time. At last we got to go there. We have always talked about it, but only it seemed as a dream. The main thing was being together. With Deb and Christopher. I think we all enjoyed it very much. Christopher tired out but rested. Babe really enjoyed everything, especially the trip through the desert. I enjoyed the slot machines, just like you see in the movies.

Brushing Away The Tears

Sunday April 26, 1992

We left for L.A. a little after 8. Stopped at Whiskey Pete's on the Nevada border. Had breakfast and did a few slot machines. Christopher got sick, but slept some on the way back. He was feeling good by the time we got to Deb's. He drove Deb's car home so we could have the rental car Monday morning. He is off Monday for his tests and stuff. A great day!

Monday April 27, 1992

Deb's going with us to the hospital tomorrow for Christopher's tests. Tonight we go to the Dodger game.

We had a good day with Donnie. He and Babe went to the hardware store and to the nursery. They planted his "big" garden. I made pictures of them. I'm not cooking today because Christopher can only have clear liquids and starts his gallon of drinking medicine at 2. We're having Dodger dogs at the ballgame. Matt went to the game with us. We had a good time but I worried about Christopher being by himself having to run to the bathroom. But he made it fine, and we left before the game was over. We have to be at the hospital by 7:15.

Thursday April 28, 1992

We left for the hospital about 6:15. I felt so sorry for Christopher because he was so hungry. I promised him as soon as he got out of there we would get him to an eating place. He was in there for 2 hours and he was weak and dizzy when he came out. We stopped at the In and Out Burgers and got him cheeseburgers, fries and a large Dr. Pepper. He was hungry all day. We went to El Coyote for supper.

Wednesday April 29, 1992

Donnie doesn't feel too good but after going through the ordeal yesterday, this is to be expected. He and Babe did more work in the garden. We are staying there tonight. Deb is taking us to the airport tomorrow so she is staying here tonight.

The verdict came in on the Rodney King trial and all hell broke loose in the Watts section of town. Couldn't sleep for police cars, helicopters, etc. I worry about Christopher living so close.

Friday April 29, 1992

How lucky we were. We left the L.A. airport at 7 a.m. Later they had to delay all flights because of all the rioting. The sky was very thick from more than 3000 fires.

Christopher wasn't feeling good so he didn't go to the airport with us. Deb dropped us off at the check in stand, so we didn't have time to cry, which was good.

Even though the garden area was very small and not very fertile, it proved to be somewhat of a success.

Handwritten letter to Mom and Dad from Christopher, June 17, 1992

A Clinic Letter

Dear Mom and Dad,

As agreed I'm sending back some of the pictures (from April). They turned out fantastic. I wish you could see my garden now. I'll have squash next week. My radishes never did do any good though. The green beans are looking great and climbing like crazy. Next year I want to plant even more. Can you believe it? I would have never thought I'd ever want a garden, out of all of us kids, I didn't like garden work. Thanks Dad!

I'm sitting waiting on my Dr. Appt. I was supposed to come Thursday, but I got sick at work and almost passed out. Then my face broke out with what looked like hives, so here I am. I think I may have had an allergic reaction to something. I've been feeling great and my appetite and energy levels have both been good. I gained a pound and a half since the last time I weighed. Yea! I don't know if I told you or not, but they suspect I may have another parasite. Yes. To tell the truth I hope so in that they can treat this stomach problem. I've been having diarrhea again. Enough of the health problems.

So it's hot and humid there? That's one thing I don't miss about the South. Now there are a lot of things I do miss, but the weather is not one of them.

After seeing the video I was terribly homesick. I have to tell you I love that duck Lola got for me. Is there any way I can have it sent? Let me know.

Katy's visit has been wonderful. I just wish she could stay longer. It seems like I never get enough of being around her. I was telling Matthew that when I'm home we spend all our time together. Lucky me. She's the perfect houseguest. I took lots of pictures and I'll send you some later.

Well, I'm getting close to the end of my paper. I love you guys so much!

Love, Christopher

P.S. I finally put my pink flamingos in the garden as well as my whirly-gig that Bobby Sue gave us. They look great. I took photos so I'll send you some.

Letter to Mom from Christopher

Tuesday, July 4, 1992

I went to my new Dr. and I feel so relieved. I think some good things might start happening now. In addition, I saw the optometrist and am getting new glasses. All in all it's been a good day.

A TEASPOON OF HOPE HELPS THE MEDICINES GO DOWN

As the summer of 1992 wore on, Christopher's journal entries were filled with his growing concern and fear that his illness was getting progressively worse. There was one bright spot in the summer – he had passed the three year pre-existing point with his insurance coverage. He could now go to a number of specialists – some of the best in the nation.

One of the nurse practitioners at Harbor Medical Center told Christopher (before the following entries) that all they could do for him was to control the pain. This devastated Christopher and caused him, as well as those who loved him, enormous mental anguish. Ultimately, I guess she was right. However, it was not acceptable to attempt to take away Christopher's hope and the fight that he was still waging with AIDS. Her words and actions continued to cause him much anguish until the end.

As you will see Christopher's new doctors never gave up hope and fought his multiple conditions aggressively and whole-heartedly. They were not about to give up as long as Christopher wanted to fight. And fight he did!

NEW JOURNAL

July 10, 1992

Handwritten

Off to see my new Doctor. Dr. Young. I feel good about this. Maybe this will be so long to Patty Cox. This could be a major turning point. I just hope I can remember everything.

A new journal and a new beginning. I know this sounds corny, but it's true in that I saw my new Dr. today. I think it's going to work out well. It will be definite improvement over my current option of the County. I still get furious when I think about Patty Cox and her, "Well, there isn't much we can do for you except give you something for the pain." That was unforgivable. I still have to deal with her this next week. I guess I'll be able to do it. We have to do what we have to do.

Saturday, July 11, 1992

It rained this morning! They have the Lotus Festival in the park today and tomorrow. No painting this weekend because of the rain. I was all packed and ready to go to Echo Park to paint during the festival.

Monday, July 13, 1992

Here we are back at the old ranch. I feel pretty good. I do feel the stomach pain coming on and should probably take codeine.

Handwritten

Hot! Hot! Hot!

Group is tonight, but I'm just not up for it.

Monday, July 13, 1992

This day has moved on slowly, but productively. I must say that I did have one energy low, but I think it was due to the Halcyon I took last night. I always have a hangover from those things. Sometimes out of the clear blue I get so sleepy. I won't get started on the physical thing.

Hopefully, I'll get to paint some tonight. One can never tell about these things. I'm having a difficult time concentrating at the moment. It's this visual thing. I hope it starts to get better and not worse. I just hope Dr. Young will be able to help.

Tuesday, July 15, 1992

I have my practitioner's appointment Thursday. I need to call today and see about having my records transferred. I'll feel so much more comfortable when I'm under the supervision of a real Doctor. I'm really concerned about this abdominal pain. The codeine makes me almost not aware of it, but I know it's there and not getting any better. Let's pray it's not anything serious. I need to go and lay down for a few minutes.

Wednesday, July 15, 1992

I'm taking off tomorrow. I have clinic, and I have to take Matthew to the airport.

Brushing Away The Tears

I might as well say it. I've been feeling very sick last night and today. Upset stomach. I threw up last night before going to bed. I felt like it this morning, but managed not to. I took two codeine today and I'm feeling better. Actually, I'm feeling sort of hungry. I'm having major thrush again. It just seems not to want to go away. I have clinic tomorrow and maybe, just maybe, they will do something about it.

Deb is going to clinic with me tomorrow. This is great in that I hate going alone. Now the drive won't be so bad. Going to Cedars is much more convenient. I hope this new Doctor works out. It's a lot of change, but hopefully it's in time. I think my luck ran out with Harbor. It's terrible, but they helped me as long as I didn't get sick. This was a terrible blow. Thank God I have another option at hand, so many don't. I still have to say that life has been very good to me. I'm just not ready for it to end. I've worked so hard to get here, and now I would like to enjoy some of the fruits of my hard labor. I know it sounds corny, but I've suffered to get where I am and now this is trying to take it all away from me. It's always been this way. I've struggled and struggled and feel like I should get a break. I have a wonderful relationship, and my art is going in a great place. With these two wonderful things in my life, why should health have to be the major issue in my life? As usual, I'll just have to cope and hopefully, as in the past, I'll overcome this. If not, then I will at least be able to say I gave it my all and tried. There are some things that are just bigger than us, and maybe this is one of them. I know I've thought that about other things, and I was able to overcome them, so maybe, just maybe, this will be the same. I certainly hope so. Life continues, and I'll try to live each and every moment. I just don't want to suffer. Is this asking too much?

Handwritten

Time for bed. Threw up my dinner and ice crème and Ensure. Boo, hiss!

Handwritten

Thursday, July 16, 1882

CLINIC

Flu – (Thrush)

Imodium

Zanax

Halcyon

Crème for rash

Anti-viral

Blood medications

Rafapin?

Throwing up

Well, it's that time of month. Could be my last visit to Harbor. Let's hope so. This is definitely a new beginning.

**Footnote - During the annual Lotus Festival at Echo Park (near downtown Los Angeles), Christopher began his last and most ambitious painting. It was a very large canvas depicting the beauty of Echo Park during the beautiful Lotus Festival. He started with a much smaller study, and in late summer then worked on the main canvas. The Lotus Festival painting seemed to become a symbol for the battle Christopher was waging with AIDS. As long as he could work on it a little every day, he felt he was making progress in art and in his fight with AIDS. The magnitude of the canvas represented the enormous task Christopher faced in "completing" this fight for his life. The goal ever present in his mind, was celebrating the day when he finished the painting, and knowing that if he finished the painting it would mean he was winning the war in his fight with AIDS.

Those of us close to Christopher knew deep down that he was unlikely to ever finish that painting but we, like Christopher, wanted to believe with all of our hearts, that it was possible. And in believing in that possibility, we all received strength from hoping that we would all be by his side when the dream of completing that painting became a reality.

Our cousin Greta did a similar small study of the same scene. She later gave her painting to me as a gift and it hangs on my living room wall today. It remains a cheerful reminder of the weekend when I observed two gifted artists at work. Somehow, I knew the moments of watching Christopher paint were limited; and that I would treasure that weekend in my memory forever.

**ptember 17, 1992*

Well, I survived Clinic yesterday. I had to miss work.

Matthew is in Wisconsin till Sunday and Greta arrives tomorrow. It was sort of nice being alone. I wouldn't want to be alone all the time, but I did enjoy the evening.

I'm now off all medications. I'm a bit nervous about this, but I'll try it; and I think it will be good to detoxify for a few days. Lots of water Christopher.

The painting is going great. I managed to get down to the park and paint for an hour or so. It's at the point that I can actually work on it in the studio as well.

I missed an important meeting yesterday. This was so disappointing. Can I maintain my job? Patty Cox thinks I should quit. No way, not right now anyway. I think she is evil. I just hope she doesn't kill me before it's too late.

** Footnote - The following is one of my favorite entries and I treasure the photos I snapped during the special weekend described in the following entry. It was the last really fun weekend I remember that we shared.

Monday, July 20, 1992

I did manage to get quite a lot of painting done. I think I'm almost ready to start the big canvas. Matthew thinks the fountain needs a little work and maybe it does. I'm really happy with the way this canvas turned out. It was a happy experience. I think I can now move outside the studio. The crowds that gathered around didn't bother me nearly as much as in the beginning. The painting works though. I must say that this Lotus painting was bottled up inside me for quite a while. I really gave this one a lot of thought. Now to transpose it to the large canvas. Greta went with me Saturday and

Sunday and I really enjoyed her company. I do wish she could have finished her painting; but alas, two days is not enough, especially in this hot weather. I think Greta could be a good painter, especially if she would keep at it. She, like me, needs more time to devote to her art. When working on something like this Echo Park Painting, I actually think that I could make it as an Artist. If I just had the chance of working for a few months uninterrupted. It's an ideal and who knows, I may have my chance. I just hope it's under favorable conditions and not related to health.

My energy level was good this weekend. I did throw up a couple of times and the rash is giving me hell. I barely can control but so far I've kept it under control. The horrible thing is that it has spread to my face. It will go away and especially now that I'm concentrating on that area with the crème. As a matter of fact I should put some on now.

I'm on no medications at the moment except Flucatozol and of course the codeine and Advil. I think I may be getting addicted to the codeine. It seems that when it starts wearing off I get irritable so I pop another one even if I'm not in any pain. Is this addiction? I should really try and make them last in that I really do still have a lot of pain at times, especially when I first get up in the mornings. I'm still trying so hard to gain some weight. Three and four Ensures a day. This is difficult within itself. I think that now I'm off all those medications my system is trying to turn back to normal. I say this because there is no diarrhea. What a joy.

I'm beginning to recover from that encounter with Patty Cox. She just as good as told me that I wouldn't be getting any better. I can't buy into that, not at this point. Why is she trying to speed it along? Mean and evil is the only thing I can think of.

Tuesday, July 21, 1992

I can't believe it, but I went to sleep for 14 hours last night. I've got to go down to Harbor this morning and get some more of the crème for my rash, which by the way, has really been active these past few days. Is there no joy in my life anymore? It's one problem after another. I must think positive and look to the future with hope. This is getting more difficult to do, but I have to do it.

I didn't work on the painting at all last night or this morning. I was too busy sleeping. I'm so pleased with the way the small study turned out. I'm really excited about getting the larger canvas started as well. At least I can do it in the studio where I have a little more control over my environment. I just need more time to work on it. I'll find the time.

Wednesday, July 22, 1992

I feel reasonably well and fairly energetic. I've just got to make it through these next few weeks. Then it's on to Dr. Young and hopefully maintenance. This pain in my abdomen still hasn't gotten any better. I still have to take the codeine and Advil. The scary thing about it is they're not trying to find out what's causing the pain any more. Assholes.

I prepared the large canvas this morning. As Matthew was leaving he said he loved the colors on the small study. This always makes me feel so good. I need that adulation. I know that little Echo Park painting is good, but it really helps to hear it. Hopefully, I'll get the drawing down and the under painting done and then it's on to the main event. I'm really excited about this painting. It's been a long time coming, but I think it's going to be worth the wait. We shall see. One never knows till it's down on the canvas.

Later...

I'm drinking my third Ensure of the day. I'm going to try and do 5 a day for a few days. I want to gain this weight back. I intend to gain this weight back. I will gain this weight back.

Christopher was remarkable in so many ways. He didn't think he suffered well. His journal entries were the only place he really admitted how sick he felt, how much he feared death was stalking him and how very scared he really was.

I remember thinking how in denial he was about his illness. But after reading the journals, I realized that he was not in denial at all. Christopher, however, possessed an enormous belief in hope and the power of positive thinking.

Excerpt from Mathew's eulogy:

"Surrender was absolutely out of the question where Christopher was concerned. With a combination of tenacity that could inspire and denial that could break your heart, he never stopped believing that he could and would get better; and he was without fail, appreciative of and cooperative with everyone who tried to help. He seemed to believe, despite everything, that he was blessed. This is the quality of gratitude that I believe set Christopher apart.

POSITIVELY POSITIVE OR KEEP ON SMILING

July 23, 1992

I'm so sick today. Sick at my stomach. Have been for the last couple of days, but it's getting worse. I have no recourse but to call Patty Cox as much as I hate to do so. We must do what we must do sometimes and this has to be handled. I have to force myself to eat. I hate that feeling. I did have another 5 Ensures yesterday but none so far today. I don't know if I can handle them today. I shall try. It's such an effort to eat. Can you believe it? Most people don't even think about it, but I have to constantly worry about eating enough. The rash has really flared up as well. I'm really going downhill and in a big way. I've got to get some help and now. I don't think I can wait another week. The worst thing is that I'm getting really weary of all this. I think Matthew is over me as well, or at least me being sick. His patience is running out. I guess it is sort of gross to talk about diarrhea and vomiting, but it's such a part of my life as of late that I don't think of it that way. I wish I could get away from it all for a moment, but it follows me wherever I go. There is no escape. I must gather all of my energy and give it one more heave ho. I shall and I feel positive about today.

I got the new canvases gridded up and started the drawing on the large one. The grid method is going to work great. I must do a complete drawing though; according to Caroline's advice. (Caroline was one of his art teachers.) *I worked on it for a little this morning, but my energy level sucks. Again, I am hit by this plague. I wonder how much I could have done if I didn't have to deal with this. I wonder how much I could get done if I had the energy level of a normal person. Will I ever know? I keep hoping that they will come up with something that will stall this thing and it sounds like they are getting closer all the time. I pray that they do and it will be soon enough for me.*

I guess this is about all for now. It seems that here lately I don't have a lot to say. I guess it's because most of it is negative.

** Footnote--I distinctly remember numerous days when Christopher looked so pale and weak when he got in the car with me to go to work. I began picking him up daily, as I knew he was getting weaker and weaker. I was constantly amazed at his determination. And it was breaking my heart every morning to see how his condition was deteriorating. He was talking less, as it required all of his effort just to remain awake.

July 27, 1992

Here it is Monday and here I am, well sort of. I feel half here in that I feel terrible. Nausea, mainly. All weekend something was wrong with me. It's enough to drive one crazy. I don't know how much longer I'll be able to continue like this. If only I could fix these couple of problems, but no, it goes on and on and on. I'm still losing *weight and it's an effort just to eat to maintain. I bought this Rapid Weight Gain powder this weekend, but I think it could have caused some of the nausea. I just don't know any more. It's as if the closer I get to seeing Dr. Young, the farther away it gets. Let's just hope that I can hang in there until that day. Tuesday, August the 4th. So Christopher, get in there and face the day with a smile.*

I started the under painting this morning. I hardly did anything all weekend, but decided that I'm not going to do a detail drawing. I just don't have it in me to do all those little details like the lotus leaves and lily pads. I think I can paint it much faster and more efficiently. Let's hope so. Funny thing, the smell of paint made me sick this morning. I guess I should say sicker.

It's an effort now just to walk up the steps from the street. Will it get worse? I keep praying that they will find something that will get me past this. If I can only hang on a bit longer, I think I can make it. I know they're getting closer to some new treatments. It's just a matter of time and at this point mine is running out and fast. One has to have food to survive and I'm hardly having any at all. I just can't force it or I'll throw up, so what's the point? All the time now I struggle. I'm not giving up yet as long as there is hope. This hope being that I'm getting a new doctor. If I didn't have this on the horizon, I might be inclined to give up. I think Patty Cox's indifference has made me much sicker. Why? Why? I've just got to get better. I have paintings that need to be finished.

Later that night, handwritten

I'm sick of being sick! Matthew cooked wonderful spaghetti, spaghetti – and I couldn't eat. Boo! I threw up and then ate 2 meatballs. I hope and pray this new medication works and gets me over this.

Tuesday, July 28, 1992

Good morning. Another day of struggle. This sounds awfully negative. Not a good way to start out the day, so here is some positive news. I'm not nauseous this morning, well not much anyway. I get a new medication today and hopefully it will do the trick. I know it will.

I painted last night, none this morning; but I did last night and it was at Matthew's urging. This makes me feel really good. To see him interested in my painting. The new painting is coming along slowly, but it is coming along. I did most of the green under painting last night. I don't know why it is, but I never enjoyed this part of the painting. I should in that there isn't much stress involved or decision making that has to be done. I think it has to do with the fact that I want to jump right in and start the painting. I definitely decided last night that I need larger brushes for this project.

Back to my health. I have a headache this morning. I took Tylenol in that I think just maybe the Advil could be causing some of the problems. I just hope Patty Cox gives me more codeine so I don't have to dole it out so sparingly. I do hate to suffer. I decided yesterday that I'm not afraid to die. I just don't want to suffer. I've always heard that from other people, but now I fully understand it. Why should I have to suffer? There is no reason. As of late, I've been fairly miserable. I want to blame Patty, and I know she could have probably done more; but it's just the way it is and I'm obviously a difficult case to treat. I'll just have to try and understand her position and where she's coming from. I'll try and be a bit more compassionate.

** Footnote - Christopher continued to worry about his frequent absences from work. He also, despite being so open about so many other areas of his life, was afraid and embarrassed to let his co-workers know he had AIDS. AIDS, even in Los Angeles, California, carried the stigma with it that other terminal illnesses lacked.

I go to Harbor today to get this new medication. Some more time at work missed. I hope this doesn't get to be a problem. It seems that

Brushing Away The Tears

I've missed a terribly lot as of late and probably will be missing a lot more in the future. If we were financially stable and able I would go on disability now. It would be embarrassing in that the secret would be out in the open and everyone would know for sure, as if they didn't already know. I think it's pretty obvious. As long as I don't declare it though, they can't say for sure. I just keep hoping that I can get past this current crisis and have a little longer to do some of the things that I want and need to have done. I've just got to try harder. It sounds so simple to just eat. The past few days have shown me that this is not true. When one is nauseated, one just cannot eat. I don't care how think you are. One can only hope in a situation like this. It seems like all I do is go on about my health. I'm sick of hearing about it and I'm sure you are also.

I guess I should go and lie down for a few minutes before the day gets started. Thank God for the cot room. Let's just pray that it stays unlocked. I'm not sleepy, but just a little fatigued. I'm always fatigued it seems. It takes an effort to climb the stairs at the house now, especially the outside ones. Will I get my strength back? I feel as if I can't ask Patty Cox questions like this any longer in that she will respond negatively. I know she will and I don't need to hear that kind of input. I need some positive input. I hope Dr. Young can provide me with some positive feedback. He seems like he can and I really do need this at this time. Patty as almost made me give up hope and begin to think that this is the end. Sad isn't it? I should really wish her well in that she needs it with an attitude like that. She obviously has problems and needs to work them out, just not on me. Good-bye Patty.

I COULD CONQUER THE WORLD

Thursday, July 30, 1992

I started the actual painting last night. Yea! It was nice and I'm excited. I didn't start until 9:00 and painted for about 45minutes. It was amazing to start a huge canvas like that. I was confronted with, where do I start? I started in a corner then went to another corner.

I'm so lucky that I have this time to do these entries. I don't know what for, because no one may ever even read them.

This has been a great day! Tomorrow is going to be even better. I must say that did take 3 codeines today and not because I really needed them, but because I like the way they make me feel. I've got to come off them, but I guess I should try and come off of them slowly. I'll have to see how the pain goes first, if it goes away, then I'll definitely have to detox from those things because I really am getting hooked. Oh well, I've had no choice and may still not have one. Maybe the pain will stay gone, let's pray that it does. Let's *pray, also, that my food starts staying down. It would be so nice to eat and know that my body is getting nutrition as well as calories.*

On days like this I feel that I could really get in there and try and move ahead again. I think I said earlier that I'm just going to try and maintain here at work, but on days like this I feel I could conquer the world, or at least, try. Adieu until tomorrow.

Friday, July 31, 1992

I made it through this week. There were a lot of good things that happened this week. I'm feeling better. The painting is starting to shape up, and I see my new doctor next week. Things are looking up. I've got to keep this positive attitude up.

I prayed again last night. It's sort of like meditation. It's reassuring in a way as well.

The painting is moving along. It's not going fast, but it's so overwhelming. I'm trying to work the canvas as a whole and it seems to be working.

It was so nice having a huge appetite yesterday and not throwing it up. My body was so grateful for the nutrition. I've had a fairly good appetite today, but not nearly as good as yesterday. I hope my experiment with taking all the drugs makes it come back full force. I must say that I do have a lot of joy in my life despite everything.

Take last night for instance. It was wonderful. We had a great evening together. It's the quiet times that I've come to love so much. Reading together is so wonderful. Matthew is teaching me the importance of reading. I don't read enough and I'm trying to improve that.

** Footnote - I was feeling increasingly overwhelmed and made a call home to my parents and my brothers in late July. As a result, my Dad and brother Glenn flew to Los Angeles to see Christopher and give us some moral support. It would be the last time Glenn would see Christopher.

Friday, August 7, 1992

I've been feeling ok. My appetite returned last night, and I was still hungry this morning. This is good in that I've been having an upset stomach all week. I am a bit weak today. I don't know what it is, but I hope Dr. Young will be able to figure it all out.

I had a great painting session last night. It's really different working so large. I've been working on it for a few weeks now, and I still don't have the whole thing worked over completely once.

Brushing Away The Tears

My Dad and brother Glenn are coming for a visit. They arrive today. I'm looking forward to going home for Thanksgiving. It's always such a treat to stay with Mom and Dad. I feel like I'm in a resort. Meals, clothes, everything prepared, not a worry in the world. This is nice.

I see a nutritionist Monday. I have a feeling they will put me on a strict diet. I need it and I think it will make a difference in my general health and the way I feel.

** Footnote - The following entry is another special one to me. Christopher muses about the dynamics of our family. He also made some very insightful observations about me. We had a unique friendship, and it was often hard for me to admit that he was right in his observations about me. We, like other siblings, often knew the right buttons to push with each other to get a reaction – good or bad.

One of the things I miss about him the most is knowing that he knew me so well and loved me anyway and he worried about me--always.

Mom's journal entry from August 7, 1992

Listening to the silence in my kitchen. It is so noticeable after all of the frantic activity this morning. I planned this trip for Babe and Glenn very well. As I sit here I'm thinking, "I wonder why did I encourage this?" Why put all this turmoil in my heart? Well, the answer is simple, and I really don't have to wonder about it. Christopher and Debbie needed someone from home, to be hugged and told things will turn out OK. If we could only believe that. I pray each day that my health will hold out so I can be there when I'm really needed. Maybe God will give me a helping hand. I'm going to try to be positive about being alone this week. I really need this time alone to get things straight in my mind. There seems to be a great sorrow in my heart all the time, and I know it shows in my outlook on everything. It seems as if everything hinges on what's gonna happen with Mother, Muzer and Christopher and myself.

Monday, August 10, 1992

I saw Dr. Young on Saturday and he took me off all milk products for the time being. He wants to send me to an Infectious Disease Specialist of which I have to call for the appointment today. If this no milk thing doesn't work then I'll probably have to have another Endoscopy. Let's hope this does the trick. I've felt pretty good most of the weekend. I just need more rest than I'm getting, and I'm getting a lot. In addition to Dr. Young, I see the nutritionists this week, maybe even today after work. The health saga continues as you can see.

Brushing Away The Tears

I'm going to Deb's house tonight. Do a load of laundry and visit with Dad and Glenn. It should be nice.

Caroline is coming by on Saturday to take a look at the progress of the painting. I want to have it in better shape by the time she comes. It makes me a bit nervous to have her come, but I think it would be great to have her input.

I hope my health will allow me to go to class this fall. I'm taking figure drawing again; but I've been thinking how much I would love to take sculpture, especially after reading this Matisse book on his sculptures. There just doesn't seem to be enough time to do everything that I need and want to do.

I must say that I really have enjoyed Glenn being here, and I'm hoping that I'll get to know him a little better. We were so close at one time. Families drift apart, especially when part of them moves away. Mom and I have stayed extremely close, but this is an exception. Of course she is an exceptional person, and so am I. I just wish there were more real communication. It seems like my family never talks about real things. We talk about things, but never really important issues. This has always been a problem with my family, and I'm sure it's not unique. I'm very lucky to have the relationship with them that I have, especially with Deb and Mom.

Deb, although she drives me crazy at times (not very often), we still have a very good line of communication. She tries so hard to be the sort of person that she thinks she should be. This doesn't allow much time for her to be the person she really is. I'm one to talk.

I've gone through so many changes these past few years. This illness has really changed me a lot. I'm no longer the energetic and optimistic person that I once was. I feel myself slowly being worn down. I need a positive break and time to regain my energy.

Tuesday, August 11, 1992

Bad start to this morning. I forgot my bag at Deb's house last night and it had my medications in it. I didn't have any Codeine or Advil this morning and I could barely get going. The pain was terrible. I almost didn't make it to work. After getting here I took them immediately and laid down for a while and now after 3 Advil and 3 Codeine, I'm feeling much better. Apparently I still have a problem. I hoped being off milk products would help with the cramping in my abdomen. Maybe it will, and I pray that it will; but for now the answer is no.

I didn't get to paint this morning due to the pain. I had the perfect opportunity to do so in that I went in later this morning and had more time. This is the way it is though, and I'll just have to live with that. This evening I'm supposed to go to Deb's early to see Dad and Glenn and do a load of laundry. It never ends. Hopefully this will be the last evening that I have to do the laundry. Actually, it's rather nice spending the time there with them. I do wish they wouldn't spend so much time watching TV; it's very difficult to communicate with the TV blaring away. Oh well, I guess they need the distraction.

I did get to paint a little last night, very little, but at least I did for a few minutes. This painting is going so slow. It's so big. I do hope to get the greens going so slow. It's so big. I do hope to get the greens locked in by this weekend. The lotus and lilies are taking a lot of time. There are parts of the canvas that I haven't even got to. As I said, it's a slow go.

This day is coming to a close. The workday that is. I must say that after I handled the pain it turned out to be a rather nice day. I'll get to see my Dad and brother though. I'm looking forward to that. I do hope we get to spend a little more time together. It seems so different without Mom here. She has a way of planning everything and making sure no one gets bored. She's always been that way. I used to be like that, but I've had to slow down. Sometimes I do well just to cope with the everyday routine. Here I go again with my health. I'm going to stop it right here.

WANTED – MIRACLES

Wednesday August 12, 1992

Well, it's hump day. I must say I'm in much better shape this morning than I was yesterday. I had a difficult time sleeping last night and ended up taking a Halcyon. Oh well, I don't think they do that much damage when taken occasionally.

I had a good painting session last night. I'm surprised, but it worked out. I was supposed to go to Deb's house and do some more laundry, but she offered to do a couple of loads and have them come to the house. So I had a couple of hours of painting.

I'm a little perturbed at my friend Judy. It seems that she hasn't been painting at all and she always has an excuse. How can she be a painter and not paint? I'm living proof that it can be done and if I can do it so can she.

I have an appointment with Clinical Partners this afternoon at 4:00. I think I'll be seeing a nutritionist. I have a feeling I'll be going on a diet. I need to, in that I know (for a fact) that I'm not eating properly. Speaking of eating, I threw up twice yesterday. I hope this stops. The diarrhea has stopped, and I'm sure it is due to the cutting out of all dairy. I feel optimistic today. Things are going to be turned around. God only knows it's about time.

I've had this nagging stomach nausea most of the day. It's really annoying. Today my stomach is extra sensitive. It's all I can do to keep food down. I've got to though. I can tell that my body is starving. I'm really excited about the nutritionist, because I think it will make a difference. I'm ready to start feeling better.

Thursday August 13, 1992

I'm so paranoid about my health as of late. Now I have learned that one of the symptoms of MAI is wasting syndrome. If this is so, then there isn't much that can be done about this weight thing. It's getting embarrassing to go out in public. I do, and I'll continue to do so; but I do wish I could gain a few pounds.

Monday August 17, 1992

Bad start this morning. Was very sick around 2:00 this morning and never did go back to sleep. I had a hot dog last night, and it just didn't digest. This with my stomach pain made for an unpleasant situation. I guess I'll have to give up hot dogs now.

Strange weekend. Greta was here, and I saw Caroline on Saturday. They all went out on Saturday, and I wasn't up for it so I stayed home. A wise decision on my part, but just another thing that I've had to give up.

Caroline gave me lots of good advice on my painting, but it's almost as if I have to start over. This painting is going to take a long time, maybe as much as 6 months. Do I have 6 months?

I wonder whether or not how much time I do have left. Nights like last night I really do think I'm going into the final stages. I don't want to admit it, but I feel so sick at the moment. I've got to get this MAI thing handled. I'm wasting away. Food doesn't appeal to me anymore, and I have to more or less force myself to eat. It's so sad in that I really did have some more paintings in me. I'll never get them out at this rate. I don't have enough to be remembered. This is so sad. If only I had started a little earlier, but no. I may make it yet and I'm not going to give up yet. I'll admit that sometimes I want to, but that feeling doesn't last very long. I've got to hold on just a bit longer.

I'm so sleepy right now. I wish the cot room were open, but I've already checked and it's not. I'll go and get the key later, but for now I'll have to hold out it seems.

I'm depressed. If things would only start looking a little better instead of all this never ending gloom, then I think I could get a second wind. But as of late I feel bad most of the time. As you can see just about everything revolves around my health. This is not the way it should be, but I don't' have a choice at the moment. I need a miracle at the moment. I believe in miracles, don't you? I think that something will turn up and this is why I have to hang in there.

Tuesday, August 18, 1992

Had a great meeting at Clinical Partners yesterday. I always feel so optimistic and up when I go there. I think they are going to fix me up with a therapist, maybe even Dr. Gibbs. I also met the nutritionist who seems like a really neat person, very warm. It's just that all of these appointments are really keeping me very busy.

I realize I still have a lot of anger toward Patty Cox. I really feel from the bottom of my heart that I've lost valuable time because of not only her indifference, but also her inability to cope with the situation. I can understand her not being able to diagnose the situation, but to say the things she said to me that day on the phone, that was unforgivable; and I'm suffering from it up to this day. I fight that negativity daily. Sometimes I believe her, and it really gets me down. If only she had been a little more responsive to my needs.

I'm getting the Codeine, hopefully today. The Pharmacist at Thrifty gave me a hard time, but Dorothy form Clinical Partners took care of it. It's so nice having someone to do things like that. I don't know why the pharmacist had to give me a hard time in the first place, but she did. All of this is hard enough without someone trying to make it more so.

Wednesday August 19, 1992

I'm reading a great book at the moment. Paul Monet's, "Becoming A Man". It's about life in the closet and boy do I relate. His experiences were so similar to what I had that at times I'm just blown away.

If I'm going to paint like a master, then I had better get on the ball. I've been rather lazy as of late. What with not feeling well and the heat. These are two more excuses for not doing what I should do. I'm not going to let them stand in my way.

Friday August 21, 1992

I feel pretty good this morning. I woke up at around 2:00 this morning with a very acute pain in my abdomen, but an Advil and Codeine took care of it. I've already had 4 Codeines and 3 Advil's this morning just to make the pain go away. I also have thrush again. One day of not taking my Flucatozole and back it comes. My T cells must be pretty low at this point. I pray that I can get them back up. I see Dr. Young tomorrow then the nutritionist Monday, then Dr. Raune on Tuesday. Busy week coming up, but I'm looking forward to it in that I think this will help matters considerable. I feel positive and optimistic once again. Now to start getting some results.

I've managed to have a great workweek. I got a lot done and my desk is immaculate. I really do enjoy working at a neat and tidy desk. I don't think it was messy before because I'm lazy, but I think my health was getting in the way of me doing a 100% job here. Hopefully, that's behind me for a while and I can really concentrate on doing a good job here. I'm also looking forward to getting back to the gym. My body is really looking terrible. Skin and bones, that's me. I've started looking better and I just know I'll look great in a few weeks.

Later that day…

I can't seem to shake this pain today. I've taken a lot of Advil and Codeine. Hopefully, this last round will do the trick.

Went to Chris's house for lunch. Read a little and slept. I was in too much pain to eat, but am doing so now. I actually went to sleep on *their sofa and had a difficult time waking up. I keep dragging this book out. I hate to put it down. It gives me encouragement to know that someone shares my situation out there and can put it into words. It is so sad to have spent his life in the closet and then come out, find someone, then they die and then he finds someone else, and they died; and now he's dying. Truly this book is a tragedy.*

According to Jennifer's scales, I've gained some weight. I'm sure I'll find out tomorrow at the Dr.'s office.

Tuesday August 25, 1992

No energy this morning. I went to bed early and had a good night's sleep, and still I have no energy this morning. I see an infectious disease doctor this afternoon, and I hope and pray that he can help me. I guess if this keeps up I'll go home around noon today.

Despite the energy low I managed to get some painting done last night. I worked on the green and the water.

At the moment I don't know if I'll be able to make it until 12:00. I feel so weak. God please let this pass. I'm beginning to wonder how much longer I will be able to work. Sometimes I think it would be better on me if I could just stay home and rest. I think the painting may have to be put on hold again and take care of this health thing.

It seems to be progressing again. I bring things under control, and then it's as if it comes back even stronger. I feel as though I'm fighting a wrestling match, and I've never been good at fighting.

When I was a kid, I always shied away from fights and confrontations. I think it was because my self-esteem was so low so I knew I was vulnerable to verbal attacks. All of those fears of constantly being afraid that someone would confront me; and they (in fact) did, many times. I don't even have time to be angry about it now. All I can think about is getting better. I rarely feel good these days. If I weren't so afraid of dying, I think I would just go ahead and give up. The truth of the matter is that I have things that I want to accomplish, and therefore I don't want to give up. I think this Doctor today will help give some insight into the matter; let's hope so. Deb will be going with me today. She's been so good about going with me. I think she's genuinely interested in what's going on. I wish I knew what's going on myself sometimes. I just hope this Doctor can figure it out and do something about it.

Wednesday, August 26, 1992

I saw the Doctor yesterday and I may have a blockage in my small intestine. If so, then there isn't much they can do about it. I go in tomorrow for some X-Rays to determine if this is it or not.

Deb just called, and I need to go and meet her. I had a sinking spell today, and it was a rough one. Complete energy breakdown. I didn't get to work until 12:00. I'm lucky I made it at all, but here I am, and I actually feel OK. I don't know what causes this, but I do wish I could find out and do something about it. I thought for sure I was going to die this morning.

I learned that my insurance only covers 6 therapy sessions. What a drag.

Fortune Cookie prediction: *There are plenty of promises and hope floating around you.*

Thursday, August 27, 1992

What an ordeal that upper GI was. I was there from 7:30 until after 12:00. No food either. I had to drink this barium liquid, and I was already feeling nauseas.

I took the night off last night from painting. I want to give the water area a little time to dry before I start painting some new leaves over it.

At the moment I'm very tired. I need to lie down for a while, but there is no chance of that in that I got here so late.

Brushing Away The Tears

Believe it or not I'm feeling pretty good today. I don't have a lot of energy, but then again I didn't get to eat all morning. My stamina has really gone down, hopefully, if I can put back on some weight it will help. I think I'm gaining again. God, I hope I get better. There is so much I want to do with my life. At the moment I can hardly plan anything beyond a few days at a time. It would be nice to think about the future with hope and plans. If I knew I had the time I would want to take some more art classes. Sculpture is pulling at me these days.

I just learned that New York is having a Matisse Retrospective this fall! Over 400 pieces, 300 of which are paintings. Oh God, I would love to go to this. This artist has been such an inspiration to me. Who knows, it may work out. I know Matthew has been waiting to go to New York and this would be a golden opportunity. The only thing is that I don't have any vacation time due to using it up at Thanksgiving. I guess we could go for a few days, but what a waste. I want to see the Guggenheim as well. There is so much that I want to do. I hope my health holds out. I just know it will. Got a lot of painting to do, and I seem to feed off of other painter's work. I noticed the brilliant greens in the Dego Riverra at the Norton Simon this weekend, and I came home and used it in my Echo Park Painting.

Brushing Away The Tears

I'm having one of my sinking spells. I don't know what to do except to go and get the cot room key. I could go home, but I really do need to be here and make up this time. I do need to stop getting the cot room key so often. I don't want to arouse suspicion. I probably already have, but I don't need to add to it. I got so paranoid last night about my job while I was stoned. All the time I've been taking off doesn't look good. I guess I'll make up a little here and a little there until it's all done. I must say it's been nice having Chris out of town for 2 weeks. It really gave me a chance to get all of those labs and Doctor's appointments out of the way. Somebody up there is watching over me. The thing is, I think they want me up there instead of down here. I don't mind dying, but I do mind the fact that I haven't finished my painting career. I don't want that to end. I know Matthew will be ok and so will my family, but will the painting just stop? If there is no after life or we don't come back, then is that just it? I would hate to think so. I would like to continue my growth as a painter. I've just barely arrived and now it could all be taken away from me. Can you say tragedy? All I can do is hope for the best and do what little I can in the time I have to do it in. I would like to learn to stop being such a TV bug. It seems that once I sit down in front of the TV, then that's it. It takes up that part of the evening that is so important to painting. After 9:00, forget it. It seems like when I get home I'm so beat from the workday that I'm no good for anything, but vegging out, which is where the TV comes in. I shall try harder to make a concerted effort to paint. There will always be excuses; but they're just that, excuses. We must not let not having ideal circumstances stop us. Life is never ideal. This disability thing appeals to me more and more when I think of the possibilities of painting. It would be rough for the first 3months, but then we could live on my 70% monthly income. Of course this means that I would probably never come back to work; but hey, do I want to be a painter or not? This may be the only chance that I still have of doing so. I don't want to wait until I'm so sick that I still have to take disability and be too sick to paint. I'll talk it over with Matthew and see what he says. We need money!!

I'm sitting here counting off the minutes until I can leave. It's after 4:00 and I need to stay until 5:00. This is very difficult to do in that I've had a long, tedious day. People are so lucky that only have their workday to worry about. My health is a major job in itself these days. I guess I should be grateful that it's not worse. What if I were going blind or had Karposia? This would even be worse.

Can you believe I've written two pages and I'm on the third? If I do go on disability I'll sure miss the computer. I just don't see how we can afford one if I have to be off work for a while. Miracles do happen though, and who knows? It certainly is my turn for one.

I learned yesterday that my insurance would only cover 6 sessions of therapy. What a bummer. I was really counting on going and letting some of this fear out. On the bright side there is the fact that I really don't have the time. I don't think I can carry on one more event. I've signed up for figure drawing again this fall, but if things don't improve I'll not be going.

I get new glasses this weekend. Yea! The ones I have are so inadequate and about to fall apart. I guess my contact lens days are over. Just another sad fact of this virus. I'll adjust as I have learned to do over and over. Life is pretty good at the moment. I say at the moment in that it changes days to day. Good days and bad days. As of late, there have been more bad days than good, but I think that is about to turn around.

Letter to Mom from Christopher, August 31, 1992

Dear Mom,

I just talked to Deb, and she says you are in recovery and about to be moved to your room. I'm so relieved that you're OK. I knew you would be, but I was still worried. I just wish I could have been there. I will be soon. You just can't imagine how much I'm looking forward to coming home this Thanksgiving. I guess it's because

Brushing Away The Tears

we've both had a rough year with our health. I just hope we're both much better by then.

I had a rough weekend. I was throwing up and felt weak. I've already called the doctor and insisted that I get an appointment this week. Believe it or not I'm not much better today. I guess that's the way it goes.

I wish I were there to help take care of you. I'm sure you'll be in good hands and everybody will help out. You're so lucky to have Noy and Tommy as well as Glenn and Teresa, and especially Noy because I know she'll look out for not only you, but Dad as well.

I guess soon I'll start to count the days until I come home. I guess it's a little premature, but I just can't wait. Anyway, I just wanted to say that I was thinking about you, and that we all love you so much. We are all so lucky to have such a caring and loving Mother. I mean that with all my heart. Not everyone is so fortunate to have the family we have, and the amazing thing is that it keeps getting better.

Tell everyone hello and that I'll be seeing them soon.

Love, Christopher

Monday August 31, 1992

What a weekend. I was sick most of it. No energy at all. Vomited three times yesterday alone. I finally managed to eat some macaroni and cheese. I'm not supposed to have cheese, but so far it hasn't affected me. I had to eat something.

We did the laundry Saturday and bringing it back in almost killed me. It totally wiped me out to bring it up the steps. All day I just didn't have any get up and go. Yesterday was even worse. I got very nauseous at the market and went outside and threw up. Thank goodness nobody saw me, but still it was a close call. I don't know how much longer I can function like this. It's getting more difficult to pretend and go through the regular routine of daily life. Now the Doctor is saying that the X-rays didn't turn up that much, but that the intestinal track was pretty clogged with the MAI. Can this be resolved? He asked me to make an appointment with him this week and we would go over the X-rays and discuss them and what I should do. I can feel that the MAI has progressed. Let's hope we can at least stall it or retard its growth. Lord, Lord. Yesterday before I even threw up and it was so weird. There was nothing in my stomach but bile and it burned like fire. On top of that I got dizzy and I had a headache. I thought I was going to have to go to the emergency room, but alas it passed. It really scared me at the time. I managed to drag through the day and did get a few things accomplished such as ordering my new glasses. This I am excited about and it's a positive thing.

It goes without saying that I didn't have a great painting weekend. I did manage to paint a little on Sunday, but not much. I was in the mood, but Matthew wanted me to go with him to run some errands and how can I say no to him after all he's done lately. He was an absolute angel yesterday.

Back to the painting. I think I may have decided what to do with the pond color. I think it's going to have to go darker. I've got a lot to do on this painting. God give me the energy to finish it and start another. We have a 3-day weekend next weekend and maybe, just maybe, I'll feel up to moving ahead of it.

This week shall be a good one. I deserve a good one after the hell week I had last week. I look forward to it with optimism and hope.

Well, this has been a rather pleasant day. I've managed to get some work done and I had a very pleasant time looking at my Matisse books on my break and my small lunch.

I have an appointment with Dr. Ruane tomorrow at 4:00 and one with the nutritionist in the morning. These should be rather easy appointments and not like the ones I had last week where I had to fast.

It's going to be a long day in that Matthew gets off at 2:00 so I'll be riding with Deb at 5:00. What's an extra hour?

I'm planning to paint tonight. I think if I move the TV in the studio then I'll be more apt to paint. This makes sense. I've started to enjoy cooking shows. I don't know how to cook, but I love watching those shows. I wonder what this means.

I keep getting interrupted here. I guess it is work, and this is secondary; but this is for prosperity. I wonder about that. Will these journals just be forgotten? It's difficult to tell.

Tuesday September1, 1992

Waiting. Today is my appointment with the nutritionist. Another appointment at 4:00 with Dr. Ruane. It's so beautiful here on this street. I really should do a drawing.

Fortune Cookie says: *Live, Think and Act for Today. Tomorrow May Be Too Late*

Just finished with the Doctor and the news is depressing. The MAI is progressing. I may have to have intravenous feeding. I'm glad Matthew was there.

Wednesday, September 2, 1992

What a day this has been. I had a CAT scan this morning which I was told would take 45 minutes. . . well, I was there about 4 hours. No food or drink except for that Barium stuff. Now I'm having problems with the pharmacy about my codeine again. They won't guarantee that it will be here Friday. I have thrush and I'm fatigued. I got a new drug today that is supposed to stimulate my appetite. It's called Megas. Well, it did the job, but the only thing is that I over stuffed myself and then threw up. So in essence, I haven't had any food today. Then on top of all of that, I had an attack of having to go to the bathroom on the way to work from the X-ray place. I pulled into a Taco Bell, but I didn't quite make it. I had to take off my underwear and then my suspenders broke. It was a nightmare in and of itself. I got to work and I have all these messages that Ren and Chris were looking for me. It's not been a good day, but it will get better.

I'm trying to check into this disability thing. Not only do I think it would be great for my painting, but I think it's becoming a very serious health issue as well. I almost didn't make it to work today. I was so wasted that I really didn't think I was going to make it to the office. I'm sure it was a combination of all the things that went on today, but it was not pleasant. So the bottom line here is that I probably need to go on disability now. My health is demanding it. I've got to slow down according to my Doctor. This means not working so much.

The pond color is dark. Can you believe it? I just can't seem to get it right. First, I thought it was too light and now I find it's too dark. The problem here is that it takes so long to cover that area and then to find out it was a waste of time. I guess it's time to call Caroline. I don't want to spend too much time on this area, but it sticks out like a sore thumb. I just hope I have the energy to work on it tonight. Something tells me that I won't, but you never know.

I just talked to Matthew and he doesn't sound too enthused about me going on disability. It's just that I don't think I'll be able to hold out here at work much longer. I think it all depends on whether or not they can arrest this MAI. If it keeps getting worse, then disability is in my future.

The following entry about his waiting to go on disability was especially upsetting to read. He *did* get that bonus, and it *was* enough to cover his cremation costs. Christopher's law firm was great about everything, including giving him this bonus even though he didn't make it until Christmas, at work or in life.

Thursday, September 3, 1992

I feel great this morning. I'm going to start having more mornings like this. Just a little weak, but not nearly as much as it has been in the past. This is going to be a great day.

Matthew and I discussed my disability options last night. I will definitely not go on it unless absolutely necessary before Christmas. I want that Christmas bonus. I've worked my ass off for it, and we need it.

It looks like we are most likely going to NY for Christmas! Matisse here we come. The only thing stopping us now is Greta's decision to come with us and trying to get decent airfares. It will work out. It is meant for me to see those paintings before I die. What I need to do is complete some more of my own paintings. I shall. I can't die just yet, because I have so many other things that I want to do. I'll die when I have the time.

Went to bed last night early, 7:30 or so. Tired was what I was.

The painting is again at a standstill. What with all these appointments I've been having it's no wonder. That one yesterday almost did me in again. It's just too much. Now, after a long night's rest, I feel rejuvenated. I need my rest.

Mom goes home from the hospital today. Yea! Deb's going home this weekend and I'm glad in that it will do Mom good to see her. I'll be going home at Thanksgiving. I'm really looking forward to it. I need a break from work and this health issue. I think I'll be able to do some good painting this time, because I'm there for 12 days.

This day has moved along very nicely. I don't know when I've felt this good. It's been a long, long time. This shall continue. It is about time!

I think I may get some painting done tonight. What shall I do? I guess I should work on the watercolor as it is bothering me. I don't want to lay the point on too thick though.

I'm working so much here lately. The Doctor thinks I should slow down a bit, but how? I only have one sick day, one personal day and not many vacation days so it's work and make up time all the time. I'm actually grateful that I can make up the time without having to document it to the minute like I used to on my other job. I have a great boss.

We need to go to the market tonight. I wish Matthew would go after he gets off work. It's unlikely that he will, but it would be nice. I can't really complain, because there are many days that I'm not worth a dime. This makes me feel inadequate. I'm full of guilt these days for what I've done to our family. I try and tell myself that it's not my fault, but the fact remains that it has caused extreme difficulty. It's sad. We were sailing along so great until all this, and now it's the dominant thing in our lives. Even on days like today when we can pretend that everything is OK, we still have tomorrow hanging over our heads. There is always the ever-present death thing. We don't really talk about it anymore, but we both are very aware of it. It's hard for me to deal with Matthew's anger because, although it's a lot of times directed at me, that is not usually where it is coming from. Still, I react in the moment of it and usually get mad or injured over it. I think sometimes he wants to distance himself from me. I don't blame him, but I do think he'll stand with me until the end, whenever that will be. I just don't know anymore what to do about the future. I don't even know anymore if I'll have one. A couple of times last month I really did think I was close to the end. It's really weird to think this could be my last summer, Thanksgiving or Christmas. I'm still going to hang in there and fight, but weeks like this one and last week really almost do me in.

This is sounding a bit morbid. I don't need to think like that, but these things have to be dealt with. I think about them, but still have a tendency to push them aside. No wonder in that I have to deal with this health issue practically 24 hours a day. Yes, I even deal with it during my sleeping hours.

Enough of that. I seem to have a great appetite with this new drug, but I really have to watch it. My food is definitely taking a long time to digest.

Matthew just called, and he did go to the market. That was so sweet of him. Now he's cleaning out the fridge and throwing a lot of things away. I do hope he didn't throw my stuff away. He has a tendency sometimes to go a little overboard. He wants me to make a salad tonight. Sounds good to me. I've got to somehow get this food to go through my intestines. At the moment I can feel it sitting there like a big lump. I pray that they will be able to do something about all of this MAI* mess that I've got myself into. They will, I just know it.

I wish everyday were like this. I did manage to take a nap today in the cot room. These really refresh me to the max. My poor immune system is having such a difficult time these days. I would like to find ways to boost it up a bit. I've got to hold on until there are some new breaks in treatments. I've just got to do so. I've got a lot of living to do. A lot of painting to do.

**Footnote - Reading over the last months of Christopher's life has been very difficult for me. One has to relive these moments while typing them into the computer. Many of those painful memories, so long buried, came back to me with agonizing force.

I remember in November of 1992 talking with Christopher while my Mom was visiting with us for an extended period of time because of his illness. His primary doctor had suggested we talk with him about his "wish list" for the time he had left. We delicately broached the subject, if one can delicately bring up dying to someone with a terminal illness. He liked to face things boldly, and I knew that it was important to him for us to have that talk. But it was the most difficult and emotional conversation I've ever had with anyone. I don't even remember how we brought it up; I only remember that he said, "Well, there are three things I really want to do: 1) Go home again for a visit. (This was after it was obvious he wouldn't likely make the trip home for Thanksgiving); 2) Go to New York to see the Matisse exhibits; 3) Finish my Echo Park Painting."

It hurt so much that he didn't even get one of his wishes, not one. And that made me feel like we had failed him. Logic doesn't really enter into the realm of watching someone die that you love. Logic also doesn't take away the feeling of being helpless. I know God was in control of his fate, and he had his reasons for denying him, (and us) the granting of the three wishes. And even while not understanding the why of it all, I understood that God would be the one to give him and us the comfort we all needed so desperately.

I am grateful for the doctors, nurses, friends and family that never let him know that we didn't believe he would live to see the fulfillment of those wishes.

When he couldn't make it home, home came to him. My brother Glenn visited in August, my brother Tommy in November, my niece Katy was there for almost two months to help us and my Dad and Mom were there for several weeks at a time. But he still had the yearning to go home.

We all must have something to live for in our lives. Christopher had those three goals clearly in his mind, and I don't believe he let go of that hope until the final seconds of his life.

*MAI – Mycobacterium Avium Intracellular – slow growing organism similar to organisms that cause tuberculosis. These organisms are extremely difficult to kill, especially in HIV patients with severely impaired immune systems and with T-4 cell counts less than 50.

Friday September 4, 1992

It's here at last. What a week this has been. Two weeks in a row of tedious appointments, but something must be working because I feel great again today.

I feel better than I did yesterday. This is amazing. Two days in a row. I'm looking forward to a great day today. I deserve it. This weekend should be even better. I think what's happening here is that I'm finally getting some nourishment, sure feels like it. I've really got to be careful though about eating smaller portions.

I didn't paint last night. I had the perfect opportunity to do so, but I vegged out. I think the color of the water is bothering me so much, and I am at such a loss as to where to take it that I'm temporarily paralyzed. I'm so afraid of over painting it that I have to make the right decision about the color.

I need to find a way at home to recharge my batteries like I do when I nap in the cot room. I seem to come in for a nosedive about 7:00 every workday. Then there is the thing that I've got addicted to 3 television shows in the evening: The Cooking Show, Golden Girls, and the news. God only knows these shows don't take any concentration. I find it so strange that I love the cooking shows.

Tonight won't be a good night to paint in that I have a hair appointment. I really do need a haircut. It's been about 3 or 4 months since the last one. I've started being a little nicer to myself lately. For a while there I let myself go more or less. I just didn't have the energy to deal with things like haircuts, clothes or glasses. I think this may be a good sign of better days to come.

I wish I were rich. Silly thing to say just out of the blue. If I had money I could paint a lot. Not only could I paint a lot, but also I could travel and paint. I'm saying this because of Matisse's travels involving painting. Maybe it will happen.

This was one of my better weeks in a long time. Tough as it was, I ended up feeling great. The now is what counts.

Later...

We're moving on toward going home. I threw up earlier. It was the peach and pudding combination that did it. I hate to throw up; it puts me in such a weird place. At the moment I feel a little dizzy and the physiological effects of throwing up are terrible as well. I was feeling so good about things in general this morning. There is a certain point that is so fine that if I cross it, I get sick. There is no rhyme or reason of when it will happen.

I'm being so good about documenting my food responses for Stephanie (my nutritionist). I really hope this works out with her. I don't want to go on intravenous feeding if I can help it, but if it will put the weight back on me, then I'll do it. I would like to know the details. I've got to put on some weight. It's a must! I look like hell. I shall look great again. I'm determined. I'll just have to get up enough steam to go for it again. This makes about the 5th or 6th time.

I don't have anything to do here at work. It's either too much or not enough. This makes me terribly sleepy. I'm going to bed early tonight, I can tell. Maria comes tomorrow, and so I have to straighten the house in order for her to clean it up.

This day is dragging by. I know it's stupid to wish your life away, but I do wish I were home. It won't be long though. Home sweet home. I like days where my workflow keeps me busy. These are the best in that I feel like I really contribute. The other cases are supposed to be heating up soon and this means work for all. Some of it will come down to me I'm sure. This has been an up and down month in more ways than one. First my health up and down, then work up and down, then there is the painting up and down. They can't all be smooth, but this month will be fantastic I can tell. It would be great to have a fantastic month, I mean all month every day. I used to have those in the old days. Now I could really appreciate them. I've just got to hang in there and be patient. I've got to make it until some new news breaks. Hold on is the word here.

All of a sudden I'm feeling better. It appears that my lunch is digesting. I've got to get some nutrition in my system. I need some body fat. Remember, small portions and an Ensure. Sounds like a good idea. I now have my delicious Ensure. Umm, umm. I've also decided to have some popcorn with my Ensure. Let's just hope it stays down. It shall and it will.

I hate when people whisper next to me. It makes me think they are talking about me. Paranoid, but it is rude.

I get a haircut tonight. I really need one if you ask me, but I just hate taking the time to get one. I'm letting my hair grow out again. It seems to be healthier now that I'm off the antibiotics. I'm on so many drugs at the moment that my poor old body must be having a difficult time dealing with it. I know I am.

Tuesday, September 8, 1992

Brushing Away The Tears

Long weekend over. I painted a lot this weekend. I made a lot of progress with it. I finally have just about resolved the water color problem. It still needs a little refinement, but I have the basic color down. Now I'm working on the city. This too is proving to be difficult in that it has to be subliminal to the Lotus. Also, along with the city is the sky color. In reality the sky was white/grey, but I think it should be a little more exciting than that. Anyway the painting definitely went forward this week.

I've had 5 days in a row where I felt good. I didn't throw up but once, which was last night. I knew yesterday morning that my stomach was out of whack and then sure enough, it finally rebelled and up came my dinner. I did manage to eat after that though. Saturday and Sunday I ate and ate. Small portions, but lots of times throughout the day. I finally feel that my body is getting some nourishment. My energy level is up to what it normally is, and now looking back on it I realize that part of the energy problem was that I have no fuel. I've already used all my fat reserve so now there is some hope that this will continue. I'm hoping that the new drug Dr. Ruane was talking about will arrest the MAI. I have positive things happening. I don't think I could take many more weeks like the past few weeks. They were hell. I was really considering disability as an alternative. If it comes to that then I'll do it, but hopefully it won't.

It looks like Greta will not be going to NY with us this Christmas. She still hasn't said no, but she wants to think about it. I think we're still going to try and do it. We really do need not only a 3rd party, but a 4th as well. I feel positive about it and feel assured that it will happen.

I'm going to stop some of this stress that I've been putting myself through and get on with my life. Things like vacations are an essential part of living. Matthew is so excited about the trip. We went to the bookstore yesterday and bought a NY guidebook and he's read almost the entire thing already. I think he's going to love NY. It'll be nice to experience the event with him. Love that man.

Thursday September 10, 1992

This week has really passed fast for me. It's almost the weekend again. I have high hopes for this one. I am really getting excited about the painting.

I think I'll finally make it completely around the canvas and can start at the Lotus again. I didn't work any last night. I lay down for a few minutes at 7:00, and that was it. I had planned to take a little nap, but I ended up sleeping until 6:10 this morning. I guess I needed it. The painting doesn't suffer from it, but just prolongs the finishing of it. I would like to get this in the final stages in that figure drawing starts next week, and I'll have to start to think about the semester final. I'm nowhere near finished on this Echo Park painting. I don't think even I realized what an undertaking it was going to be. Did I take on too much? I don't think so. We'll see when it's finished whether or not it will be worth it. I have real good feelings about this one and so far it's been pretty much a nice experience. Now that I'm feeling better, even more so.

I'm finally eating and getting some nourishment. Yesterday was a great eating day and today will be as well. I did wake up with a bit of pain this morning, but I'm use to that. I've already had eggs, toast, coffee and juice this morning and I'm hungry at the moment. It looks like disability will be put off for a while now. I would have had to make it until December anyway. I don't want to jeopardize my Christmas bonus. That is what we're going to NY on.

It appears that we are indeed, probably, most likely going to NY to see the Matisse's. The thought of it gives me chill bumps. I think it's like Matthew says, that I respond emotionally to Matisse in a way that I haven't in other artists, even Van Gogh. I'm trying to absorb all that I can of Matisse. I would like to experiment with some of his styles and techniques and see what happens. Even though his style seems simple, it is not. I love Matisse. Thank you Matisse for giving us so much. I hope and pray that I can give a 1/3 as much as you have to the world. That's what it's really like you know. We as artists are indebted to give to the world. It doesn't really matter that paintings are sold and profits are made left and right. The bottom line is that it's done out of a creative search and the need to say something about the world around us and who we are and how it affects us. This may sound a little mushy, but who cares? I wonder if Matisse knew the effect that he would have on people like me? Did he know that he was leaving behind a legacy? I have that feeling. I just hope that I can leave behind enough that will say something. I don't want to be morbid, but my chances of being around a long time aren't that great. Canvases like the one I'm working on take up a lot of time. I think that for the sake of output I'll work smaller next time. I haven't really tried any really small canvases. Matisse did; and if he did, then I shall.

Looks like it's going to be another one of those days when I work a little and write a little. I used to look at this as typing practice, and I guess it really is.

I'm feeling a bit dizzy and sick to my stomach at the moment. I think it could be the medications. I have to take so many of them that sometimes they don't mix very well. I wish the cot room was open, but alas, I just know it's not. If I could go and lie down for a few minutes, I'm sure this would pass. I guess I could lay my head down, but this doesn't seem to work well. Christopher, Christopher, what are we going to do with you?

I finally threw up. The only thing that came up was the mango I had last night. It seems that everything else had passed through including the eggs from this morning. I guess high fiber fruits are off my list. Last week I threw up a peach so I guess I'll just have to avoid certain fruits.

I now feel much better though. Now I have to make up for the loss of that food. The thing that concerns me is that I don't know whether or not I lost my medication this morning. I don't think so, but there isn't really any way of telling. I'll just have to take them again when I get home. Life is so complicated sometimes. This reminds me that I should really keep at least one days medication in my bag. Actually, I should keep more in case of an emergency, such as an earthquake. Things are still tasting funny. I'm drinking a regular coke, and it's terrible. I'm a mess today. It'll get better. I feel it in my bones.

Today has been a struggle. No more mangos! Adieu.

**Footnote - Most people like to believe, deep down, having money is not a pre-requisite for having a happy life. I tend to agree most of the time with that assessment. When one is faced with a terminal illness however, and worried about financial matters, being financially secure would make a lot of difference. Christopher, like most people, felt as if he had to work in order to contribute to his and Matthew's household. In hindsight it is easy to say, "Nothing should have been more important than his health." He, as most people would be, was in denial to some extent; and so he plowed on as best he could. The image of him crawling under his desk to nap, breaks my heart.

NEW JOURNAL – STILL GOING

Friday, September 11, 1992

Here we are again poised on the brink of another fabulous weekend. I think it's going to be a great one. I'll just have to admit that yesterday was fairly bad. I threw up again when I got home and felt very tired. I did manage to eat quite a lot though and my strength returned. I just couldn't shake the nausea yesterday. It stayed with me all day.

Today I got up at 5:30 to paint, and after showering I was so cold that I got back into the bed and stayed there until almost 6:30. I just could not get warm this morning. I think I may have a touch of the flu. It's been trying to come on all week, and I think it may have succeeded. I'm out of Advil so I'm having to take Tylenol which never seems to do as well. Other than this, I feel pretty good. My energy is still down a bit, but not as bad as it has been in the last few weeks. Progress I guess.

I'm at work at the moment and hopefully some work will come in.

I've just discovered that I can crawl under my desk and snooze if need be. It makes me nervous, but I'll do it if I think I absolutely have to do so.

New Journal. It's always difficult to give up the old one. I depend on it a lot to help keep me organized. I need to re-organize my journals into some sort of order. Actually, I need to straighten up the shelves in the studio. This would include the journals.

I've been sleepy most of the day, and my stomach is bothering me again. I wouldn't call it a bad day, but it's not one of my best. Sometimes all this is almost too much to take. Health and work and home life. It's quite complicated and doesn't seem to let up very often. At least we get to go home early this afternoon. This I am looking forward to and just maybe, just maybe I'll get some painting done.

I'm counting the minutes until I get to go home. This day has been a real drag. I will have this weekend at home. I love my home life. I love my man, and I love my cats.

** Footnote: Christopher's phrase, "I was really hoping I would be put back together by this time," reminded me of my own image of him as Humpty Dumpty. His loved ones teamed with his medical caregivers; and just like "all the kings men and all the kings women," we couldn't put him back together again.

Monday, September 14, 1992

Monday, Monday how I dread that day. Terrible weekend in that I was in bed for most of it. I find it difficult to believe that I had all those great days and then boom, sick. It's not fair I tell you, and I know that life is not fair; but this is really beginning to get me down.

Needless to say, I did hardly any painting this weekend. I did manage to do a little, but it almost did me in. No energy. I have class tonight and am planning to go. I really shouldn't, but would really like to do so. I was really hoping that I would be put together by this time, but alas it didn't happen. Hopefully soon, hopefully soon.

I may not have painted, but I did manage to make it to work. I am beginning to wonder how much longer I can keep this up. Not long I don't think. Maybe, just maybe, I can hang in there until November, and I am going to give it my best shot; but it's going to be a long uphill effort.

** Footnote – I remember thinking, numerous times, how it seemed as if Christopher was rock climbing and just when he would reach a handhold, fate would knock him back down. It was horrible seeing him in such agonizing pain during his hospital stays.

Handwritten

Wednesday September 16, 1992

C. Sinai Hospital . Waiting for my IV to be put in place. Jesus, what a mess. Although I feel positive about this, I just wish it had been done earlier.

Friday September 18, 1992

What a week. I have missed the last 3 days and have seen 5 doctors and will see another today. Busy, busy, busy week for me. I start my IV feeding tonight, and I'm counting the hours. No painting at all. I was too weak to hold the brush up. I did try one day, but it was impossible. Needless to say I didn't make it to class either.

I'm happy about the prospect of putting on some weight. This sounds as if it's a sure shot way to do so.

Handwritten – for the rest of his journals

Tuesday September 22 1992

Whew! A lot going on here. I'm in the hospital. Yes, it's true. I was in such horrible pain. It would not go away. Now they have me on morphine. Boy! What a trip, but it's working. I was in continual pain for 2 days. It appears that I may have to have surgery. We should know tomorrow. At the moment I'm having a difficult time focusing. It could be the drugs. I'm out of pain! Thanks God!

Long day. Not a lot of positive information. I'll fill in details later. I pray that things turn out OK. I obviously can't focus to write.

I'm talking to myself. Bad! My first watercolor was terrible. I guess I should go to bed and hope for a better day tomorrow. I'm stoned.

Thursday September 24, 1992

Well, things are looking up. I may go home tomorrow! I'm having solid food again. And they have the pain problem solved (almost solved). Mom and Dad are here. I will probably have to have surgery, but the surgeon feels good about it in that I have only one blockage and it's in an area easily assessable. So good day.

I'm getting ready for a blood transfusion. (Low Blood)

So I'm feeling great! Looking good too. I will have to be on a 24 hour I.V. for pain, but hey.

Friday September 25, 1992

Still here. More tests tomorrow. It will be positive tests, and I'll get out tomorrow. I don't think I have a second blockage. I don't. I'm happy that I think I don't. I was edgy today. The drugs, I'm sure. It's 11:00 p.m. and I should really get some sleep. Mom and Dad are here. Greta is here as well. I do hope I lose this edgy feeling.

I had 3 enemas tonight and 3 different types of laxatives. I know where I'll be tonight. Life goes on.

Mom's Journal Entry

September 26, 1992

Left for the hospital about 10 and will spend most of the day there. Christopher is going home tomorrow. I'm so worried. Deb looks so tired. God bless her.

September 29, 1992

I can't focus, so this will be brief. Out of hospital Sunday. I'm doing great! I now weigh 122. This may not sound like a lot.

Later . . .

Problems with my TPN. Waiting on the nurse to call. Which she will soon.

My pain is gone, of course I'm on 3 mg of Diludid every hour, but it's gone.

No painting as of yet. I want to give myself a few days to regain some strength, which is happening.

Mom's Journal Entries

September 20, 1992

Christopher is feeling better. Going to the hospital to get tubes changed Thursday. Babe canceled his flight and is staying longer. I'm staying here tomorrow for a medicine delivery.

October 1, 1992

Deb called and said they left for the hospital about 5:30 a.m. Got home about 2:30. Deb called and kept me informed about the procedure. A long and very tiring day. Deb went into work for awhile and got back to Christopher's about 6:30. She is really wearing herself out. We are so worried and concerned about her.

Saturday October 3, 1992

(Sorry about the handwriting, drugs you know)

I'm so stoned on the Dilaudid. Being home has not turned out the way I had expected. I thought I could rest but there is always something going on. Nurses, medication and of course all the phone calls. The phone rings constantly. It's nice, and don't get me wrong, but I've got to get some rest here. I think next week will be better. The medication the nurse is infusing will be over on Tuesday.

If I could only paint some, I think I would feel better. I've got to take advantage of this situation. So do it Christopher (sorry about the handwriting)

Notes

TPN Food bags and vitamins

TPN –CVP dressing change and tubing for TPN

Truy #1236

Battery for PCS

**Footnote - During the last months of Christopher's life, I often worked at home and at odd hours in an effort to catch up on the work I missed because of my numerous hours spent with Christopher.

Mom's Journal Entry

October 5, 1992

We're leaving for home in the morning. So today has been a sad one for us. Christopher is feeling pretty good. I hate to leave, but I've got to go home and see if I can get some help for my back.

Christopher is like a kid, so grateful we've come. Deb is pitiful too. How can I leave?

October 6, 1992

Left the L.A. airport at 7a.m. Got home about 7p.m.. So tired, upset, worried. People coming and going. Talked to Christopher and Debbie, think they are about the same. No one will ever know how hard it was for us to leave.

Letter from me to my parents

Saturday October 10, 1992

Dear Mom and Dad:

I'm sitting here at the computer at home listening to my Halloween wind chimes. I've done some work to print on Monday and still have like one or two hours tomorrow.

The future seems so vague right now. I guess that's because I still feel in a "crisis mode" and it's hard to plan beyond today. I'm grateful that things have improved over the last few days. I am trying to stay positive about things because that is "good luck thinking". Tim helped me set my room straight last night and we moved the futon out. I told him that even though one or both of you, or someone else from home, might be back soon, it is better to carry out actions as if it will not be necessary for you to come back. Maybe things will work out that way. Does that make sense to you? It does to me in a weird kind of way. As much as I love having you and/or Dad out here, I just pray things will be stable enough and Christopher will be well enough to travel home next month. I want that so much, and I know you do too.

Like we say, all of this stress and sadness does make us stronger; and if I can survive this and remain half way intact, then conquering another job search will seem like a piece of cake. It's funny and sad how things like we are going through now make everything else we've been through seem easy. I picked up and changed my life once; and when the time is right, I can do it again. I really don't want you and Dad to worry too much about me (I know you can't help it) because God is giving me the strength from somewhere to carry on. I know that 5 or 6 years ago we would have doubted my ability to go through something like this. But there is some satisfaction in reaching deep down and doing something solely for love of someone else and from the depths of your heart. I am sure the reason I'm finding the strength also is because of the way you and Dad raised us. Things like that are not really learned later in life. I pray every night that I don't lose it! I really don't think it is something you can lose. It was really hard not to stop myself from begging you and Dad not to go but I'm glad we all found the strength to see what was sensible and necessary. It would have been selfish of me to put you in that position.

Tomorrow I will take Christopher's laundry home (just 2 small loads and I didn't fold them as well as you!). I was going by today, but Gina stayed 2 hours; and he is worn out from his vacuuming frenzy, so I will give myself a break today too. I want to see him, yet I welcome the necessity of not going. Does that sound bad?

Thursday night (Christopher's birthday) Jeff and I have a screening at NBC, and we get dinner and $20! I plan to take a long lunch and take Christopher's things to him and spend a couple of hours with him. Unfortunately, we can't all have champagne and dinner anyway. Maybe he and Matthew can have a pleasant few hours alone Thursday night. I think I will get them two nice candles for the occasion.

Debbie

October 11, 1992

What a strange weekend this has been. For once I did not worry about having so little time. Tomorrow is a new workweek, and I must define it. I'm going to need energy in the morning.

My notes from October 12, 1992

TPC Nursing

Janica 800-366-4872

Will be talking to Dr. Geenfield. Norelle Nursing Service to evaluate. Will be out here to evaluate.

Mom's Journal Entry

October 12, 1992

Talked to Christopher. He had a bad night. We may have to go back any time. He can't have anything to eat. Deb spent the day with him, afraid to leave him by himself. Debbie is really scared. He is hallucinating, on so much medicine.

Wednesday October 14, 1992

Deb called and was really upset. God bless her, she has so much on her plate.

**Footnote - On October 15, 1992 we celebrated Christopher's 39th birthday. It was very difficult to be in a festive mood. We knew that it was important to focus our energy on making sure it was a good day for Christopher. My parents had returned to Alabama after Christopher's September hospital stay. My mother had to attend to my grandmother, who had leukemia and was in the early stages of Alzheimer's as well. I remember going to Christopher's house for lunch and taking him cute bunny boxers and some roses. I don't remember now what Mom had sent him. She was always sending us great care packages.

As he became increasingly ill, his journal entries were more sporadic and the effects of the drugs were obvious in relation to his writing abilities.

Mom's Journal Entry

October 15, 1992

My mind is in L.A. wanting to be with Christopher. Tom and Glenn talked with him a couple of times. His birthday is today.

October 16, 1992

3:00 a.m. Legs numb, short of breath. I called. Doug was on call. He told me to put the pump in, stop and turn it back on in the morning for a couple of hours. What can I do? Oh well,

Brushing Away The Tears

The following was a list of issues important to Christopher on the ballot for voting. Voting was very important to him and he voted, in the 1992 Presidential election, absentee as well.

Prop 167, Supervisor - NO

Borrowing from next year's funds no

Adopted Budget

12 libraries closed

1,000 people laid off

Closing jail cells

Fees for special services

Horse Trails

Bike Trails

Golf Courses

Museums

County cuts

October was filled with our family's birthdays. My 32nd birthday was Sunday, Oct. 25, 1992. Christopher believed in making everyone's birthday a wonderful, special event. He was great at choosing just the right gift for the personality of the person celebrating the birthday, anniversary or other special occasion. He made the monumental effort of shopping for my birthday that year. He bought me pearls and a hat. He said even though he knew that I was not a hat person per se, he felt every girl should own at least one hat. He made a big deal out of the presentation of the gifts as well. I was so excited to see the huge wrapped box and colorful bags. Deep down, I was afraid this would be the last birthday gifts I would ever receive from him. It turned out to be his last shopping trip as well.

Mom's Journal Entry

October 26, 1992

Deb called and told us Christopher is back in the hospital. I went to physical therapy but was so upset they sent me home. My God, what will we do? Please God, let things get better for him. I love him so much and please help Deb too. It is so much for us to bear. I'm glad Katy is there with them.

Saturday October 31, 1992

Well, here's a catch up.

Back in the hospital. Yes, I've been here since early Monday morning. Horrible pain. That Dilaudid wasn't taking care of it either. But, and this is a big but, I may not have MAI as suggested. This is the most wonderful news in a long, long time. They're getting closer to what the problem is and here it is. I have Pancreatitis (an inflammation of the Pancreas). This is causing pressure against my intestines. This could be caused by several things. I could have gallstones which could be removed with little trouble. I may have to have my gall bladder removed, which they can now do and not leave but a tiny scar. There still remains the issue of the swollen lymph nodes. These can also be removed with little trouble and little scaring. So things are looking good. Not just good, but great. So I'm feeling good. Bored, but I am getting much better; and this is what counts. I've had my pain medication reduced from 35ml to 20ml an hour.

**Footnote - The roller coaster continued with a different diagnosis daily. Such is the nature of full-blown AIDS. The immune system is so compromised that it is confusing to know all of the things happening in the victim's body. Remember, none of us had experience of the up close and personal side of this disease until

Brushing Away The Tears

Christopher's HIV diagnosis. Like Christopher, we would get our hopes up only to have them dashed as another problem popped up.

On a lighter note, the employees of the Sixth-floor at Cedars Sinai dressed outrageously for Halloween that year. It really cheered up Christopher and the other patients. Christopher and I shared a great love of the fun of Halloween.

In the middle of all of this sadness, I was working on the most exciting project I had been involved in since moving to Los Angeles. It seems most people dream of working in or around the movie business. I kind of stumbled into the job of location filming coordinator at the Westin Bonaventure Hotel. During the summer and fall of 1992, I was working with the location manager and production staff for the filming of numerous scenes for the movie, "In the Line of Fire," starring Clint Eastwood. I truly believe that project helped me keep my sanity intact as I had to focus a lot of energy on making sure the hotel's commitment to the movie cast and crew was honored. Kokayi Aamph was the location manager and Martine White (the former film commissioner of Santa Barbara, California) was the assistant location manager. The two of them became friends and provided understanding and comfort to me during the pre-filming, filming and post-production of "In the Line of Fire." Everyone associated with Castle Rock Productions and the film was so understanding and helpful. I remember reviewing the lengthy contracts between the hotel and the film while at the hospital with Christopher. I took solace in reading the legal jargon as it kept my mind totally focused and provided a brief escape from the cloud of illness swirling around my family and me.

The night before his surgery I was at the hospital with Christopher for a few hours alone. It was rare that we had any time alone since his first hospitalization. When we were alone he was sleeping much of the time. I was terrified that he would not make it through the surgery. Mom had gone home for a week or so to take care of my grandmother. I was feeling so overwhelmed with fear, sadness, and anxiety. Christopher was able to walk a little, and he came to me as I stood at the window in his room, crying but with my back to him, because I was fighting so hard not to let him see me cry. He put his arm around me and he said, "Please let it out. It's okay, Deb. You are supposed to cry to your big brother. That's what I'm here for." And cry I did.

For a long while I cried on his shoulder, for the first time in a very long time. Just like I did when we were kids and our other brothers were picking on me, just like I did as a teenager when some boy had hurt my feelings, just as I had done as an adult because of a disappointment. When I had cried myself out to the point of hiccupping like children do when they cry too much, he started to cry softly; and he said, "That's one of the things I've missed the most during this nightmare, is taking care of you and providing comfort for you, and knowing that I'm causing you all of this pain."

As painful as that was, I am grateful that we had that special time together. In many ways we did get our chance to say goodbye to each other and to visit, one last time, that unique bond that had existed between us since my birth.

Room 6820, November 1, 1992

Sunday November 1, 1992

Well, I'm feeling better every day. Soon, just maybe I'll be able to eat again. One never knows how much one misses things until they don't have them. I've been without food for so long and I miss it.

Monday November 2, 1992

Election tomorrow!

I'm rather sleepy at the moment.

Goodnight.

(Christopher loved to play Backgammon and we played a lot during his hospital stays.)

Mom's Journal Entries

Thursday, November 12, 1992

Deb called. Christopher is in ICU. Received tickets on Northwest to leave tomorrow morning. God, please save him. We need your help.

Friday, November 13, 1992

Jeff picked us up in Burbank and we went straight to the hospital. Christopher is still in ICU. He looks so terrible. I'm happy I am here, feels so good to hold him in my arms like he was my little boy again. Stayed at the hotel with Debbie and Katy. Debbie is staying here for the filming of, "In the Line of Fire" with Clint Eastwood!

Sunday November 14, 1992

I haven't written anything in over a week. I'll make Quic.

Tuesday – *we won all around.*

Wed – scheduled for a liquid from stomach. The older doctor came in and I proudly showed him my stool and vomit. He instantly went to the front desk and it was hell from then on. I.C.U., 6 pints of blood. This was blood the Dr. had looked at then performed the endoscopic procedure that night (morning), 4 liters of blood from my stomach they removed. Yuk! I stayed in ICU all day and moved here.

Oh yeah, I forgot to mention on Wednesday I had my surgery. The worst pain I have ever had in my whole life.

Now, I have 21 or so staples up my sternum. Upped my pain medication 25mg an hour. I saw the surgeon on Saturday and he said I was his miracle case. Now, it's Sunday night. I've gone back up.

That was Christopher's last entry in a lifetime of journals.

Mom's Journal Entries

November 15, 1992

Stayed at the hospital for several hours. I feel so helpless. Deb is so tired and it shows. I'm glad I'm here. It's so hard on her driving to work and to the hospital in all the traffic.

November 16, 1992

Deb drove me and Katy to the hospital, then went to work. Christopher seemed very happy we were there. Katy is really great with him. I feel so helpless. I fixed our breakfast before we left. It's so hard leaving him.

November 17, 1992

I spent all day at the hospital. No one knows unless they have been through this how it hurts to sit and know your child is sick and not going to be well ever again. I've cried till it hurts, but it doesn't help.

November 19, 1992

Spent the day with Christopher. Tommy is coming tomorrow. Katy is working at the hotel. I'm so worried about my mother also. God, just let me hang on.

November 20, 1992

Tommy arrived! Yea! Jeff and Katy picked him up at the airport. We went to he hospital after Debbie got home. I'm renting a car in the morning. Will cost a lot but will help Deb so much. I don't know what we will do when our money is gone, but it's going fast. I thank God Tommy is here. He was really shocked at seeing how sick Christopher is and how much weight he's lost.

**Footnote - Christopher was in the hospital until the day before Thanksgiving. Mom, meanwhile, came back to visit for more than a month. Our niece, Katy, came on Oct. 24th to help out and to give me moral support. Dad came back for several weeks, and our brother Tommy came in mid-November and stayed through Thanksgiving. My roommates, Jeff, Brian, Tim and David, rallied around us and willingly gave up space in our rental house in Burbank to my family members. They also handled numerous daily chores and tasks for my family and me. I was so fortunate to be surrounded by unbelievable support. Additionally, my friends Tony, Kevin and Christine gave me enormous emotional support daily. And they made me laugh when there was little to laugh about. Sometimes I think that was the thing that kept me sane during that very difficult period of my life. Tony was always reminding me that I shared Christopher's wry sense of humor and that I must use it to get me through.

Two days before Thanksgiving, Christopher's doctor called me out into the hall alone. Mom, Tommy and Katy were in the room with Christopher as I exited to speak to the doctor. The doctor had that intensely grave look that no one ever wants to see. He said that in his estimation, Christopher only had a few weeks to live and that he was sending him home with all of his medications, home health care, etc., so he could be with his family during the last part of his life. He said it was up to our family to decide what, if anything, we would tell Christopher. I fought harder not to sob uncontrollably than I've ever fought in my life because, right or wrong, we would not be telling Christopher this latest news. Not that it was news to him, I realized after reading his journals. But I'm sure I wasn't really hiding anything anyway. He knew me too well. And I'm sure the look on my face when I returned, smiling through my tears, told him what we were all too scared to say. Instead, we focused on the only bit of good news we could. He was finally coming home.

Mom's Journal Entry

November 24, 1992

Bad News! We waited until Deb got home to go to the hospital. Dr. Ruane talked with Deb. Said Christopher is not going to make it. He's not doing any good. My God, what a nightmare. I can't believe it, but in my heart I knew. Tommy was our salvation. We could not have gotten through this night without him. I pray that Deb can come to grips with it. I've got to hold up for her.

Brushing Away The Tears

**Footnote - After we left the hospital, I finally was able to sob out the details to the family of what the doctor told me. Though I tried to hold back knowing that my mother, Christopher's mother – was in this small audience in the car. Indeed, she was heartbroken. Torn between knowing it was near the end for her second born son and trying to comfort her daughter after hearing the most devastating news, to date, of her life. The conversation I had with the doctor that terrible day was the first time we had actually been given any sort of time range. The doctor chose me, because I had been involved in Christopher's case from day one, and he also said he really couldn't bring himself to tell our mom.

When we finally reached our house in Burbank, it was plain that Tommy was also torn up about the news I had delivered. He kept hugging me and telling me how we have to hang on to hope, but at the same time to start letting go in order not to have a complete meltdown. He said that it is all in God's hands now, and we had to accept what may come next. He also recounted a heartbreaking story of a loss of a buddy he suffered while serving in the Air Force during Vietnam. He said God takes care of you when you absolutely think you can't bear the trauma of losing someone about whom you care.

I felt that God was preparing all of us for what was to come. I can't imagine how people cope when the loss is sudden and unexpected. In our case, there were months of moments and actions of saying goodbye. And God sent me my family when I needed them the most. He sent me challenging work to keep me from having the luxury of falling apart.

Homecoming proved to be a nightmare logistically. The main part of Christopher's rental house was up 33 stairs. Thankfully, Tommy was with us and assisted with getting doors off of hinges, etc. to bring him in on the stretcher. But the joy of knowing that he made it home was a milestone in itself, and so we were truly thankful during Thanksgiving 1992.

At my house in Burbank, as usual, a large feast was being organized with a lot of our friends invited. Family was in town and no matter what was happening, the great Southern tradition of thinking food would cure any illness or sadness continued.

November 25, 1992

Tommy, Katy and me took Deb to work and we spent the day at Deb's. I went to the market to get stuff for Thanksgiving. We went to the hospital and then came home and waited for Christopher to get home in the ambulance. He was so cold and tired. I'm so happy he is home. They did all they can do for him at the hospital. He won't be able to come to Deb's for dinner tomorrow.

November 27, 1992

Spent time with Christopher. Did laundry. Packed our bags to stay at the hotel and Christopher's this week. Deb hates to be at the hotel this week but has to be on call. I feel so bad for her.

**Footnote - After Thanksgiving, work was very intense for me. Katy and I moved into the hotel for several weeks while filming, "In the Line of Fire." It was also closer for me to Christopher's house. I had to work a lot of nights and slip off when I could to visit my brother.

My Mom stayed until Dec.7. Things were getting worse for her at home with my grandmother, and she had to leave Christopher and me for a while. When she left Christopher was doing better and was even able to read and receive visitors. I dropped her off at the airport that morning before work. I battled the strong desire to pull her back and beg her not to leave. I had to face work and another rigorous day of filming, so I had to hold my fear and emotions at bay. Work had to be done.

Mom's Journal Entries

Brushing Away The Tears

December 8, 1992

On the plane. Guess I'm out of Los Angeles by now. It's lonely traveling alone. My heart is still aching so much. I can hardly wait to have Babe's arms around me so I can cry my heart out. Although I don't think I will ever get rid of all the tears inside of me. Never. Never. But life goes on. I'm so glad Deb came back this morning at the Burbank airport, for the last hug is always the best. I love her so much. I pray for Christopher and that he stays well long enough for Deb to enjoy her visit home at Christmas, and I pray that Christopher will get to come home soon. Please God, let this be so. A very tiring day, heart wrenching to leave Christopher and Deb.

Got home at 11:30. It was so good to be in Babe's arms and to be in my home. I'm so sad that I had to leave. Life will be hell for me. Felt so good to be able to cry and to have Babe's hugs and Noy and Tommy's hugs. But how will I stand being here when Christopher is dying so far away?

**Footnote - Katy was with me until Sunday, December 3rd. During her last morning in Los Angeles we decorated Christopher's Christmas tree. We helped him down the stairs from his bedroom. He watched as we decorated the tree and reminisced about the origin of many of the ornaments. Christopher loved decorating the tree, and we have video of him decorating their tree in 1991 that I treasure.

I dropped Katy off at the airport waiting area and actually went back to get her several times to say, "You can't go." We are going back to the hotel because I can't bear to face this alone. But I knew her family was missing her. She had been with me for almost two months. Also, the thought occurred to me that I didn't want her to see Christopher suffer anymore than she already had. She was wonderful with him and became a pro at changing bandages, preparing his IV and pain machine. It was now time for me to be the grown up and let her go.

Mom's last letter to Christopher

December 10, 1992

Hi and a big hug from Alabama. Gosh, I miss you. Hope you are having a good day. I've been busy, busy, busy since I returned home. I'm at Lucy's (her hairdresser) and it feels great to be under this dryer.

I really have missed taking care of you these last few days. You are always in my thoughts day and night. I love you and will see you again soon. I'm glad you have Charles (his home health nurse) during the day. He seems to be a kind and loving person. I like him. Take care. We love you and pray you will soon be able to come home for a visit. Maybe when the tulips are in bloom, if not before then.

Love Mom

The last day of filming for "In the Line of Fire" was Monday Dec. 14, 1992. It was a hectic day with major scenes being filming. At the end of the successful shoot, I was fortunate to have my picture taken with Clint Eastwood! I was thrilled and exhausted, but that picture made it all worthwhile!

As a result of the long, stressful hours I had maintained during the filming, I asked to be off Thursday, Dec. 17. My boss tried to get me to withdraw the request because there were so many things going on at the hotel, and she would be out of town and needed me to cover the office. I insisted that I was exhausted and really needed the down time to prepare for Christmas and my trip home (although I knew I probably wouldn't get to go home, because I couldn't leave Christopher). So she granted my request.

I spent several hours on Tuesday and Wednesday evening at Christopher's. He was weak and did not return downstairs after our tree trimming. His friend, art instructor and mentor, Caroline Blake, visited him during the day on Wednesday Dec. 16th. The following is an excerpt that she wrote about her last visit with Christopher.

"Over three years I've watched Christopher blend new skills and concepts into his own emerging abilities in drawing, color and design and painting classes. From our very first drawing class at Otis Parsons, he was serious and disciplined, determined to work through difficult stages. Christopher progressed and eventually came to hold his own, earning the respect of other classmates. He would rise very early to paint for an hour before work, revealing the view from his window. He started an exchange of artworks among students, sort of a rotating non-rental gallery. I am told he sacrificed his wardrobe budget to buy the best in art materials.

His homage to Van Gogh project happily coincided with a flight to Amsterdam and a pilgrimage to Van Gogh's home and a viewing of the international celebration of that artist's 100th birthday. He warmly embraced his friends from class on his return, and they adored. him. We all did.

After our classes together ended in 1991 there were three more painting class reunions and a memorable party in his hospital room in September (of 1992). And as several of us scattered, there were the telephone calls amongst the group, tracking Christopher's condition. And he phoned us periodically, full of gentle interest, intent on urging everyone to maintain and push their drawing and painting skills.

One morning last summer, while I was confined to my bed with a mild concussion, Christopher phoned me about was to be his largest and most complex work to date – the Echo Park canvas for which he did preliminary smaller drawings and color studies. I was amazed to hear myself willingly and coherently confer with him. He told me while on location in the park he was surrounded by curious on-lookers and would be art critics. His impetus was to tackle even more demanding projects, a needed reminder during my own faulty condition, of the persistence of joy and the physical inconveniences the spirit is equipped to defy. And as I relinquish myself to the fact of his death, I take solace in recalling his total involvement and in the joy of his work.

Some viewers may find Christopher's self-portrait with concertina wire disturbing. It is a depiction of a universal condition, a subject interpreted by Goya as well. Completed within a short time frame last summer, it is a powerful work which compressed his growth, restructured his handling of brushstrokes, varied his paint pressures, clarified his figure drawing skills and transformed his pain into art. In it, he moved away from a depiction of the surface beauty of nature, seen in his more frequent landscaped and away from the sensuality and comfort of color which was often his forte. Its starkness depicts a dark place of the soul, Christopher's Gethsemane, caught between darkness on one side and daylight on the other, it is a portrait of silent horror made specific. Christopher was very excited about approaching this work again after leaving Michael Wingo's studio. There he and Michael, a respected painter and Otis instructor, spent an intense hour or more discussing the significance of this work and how best to approach it.

Insistently, as an acolyte, Christopher moved away from the trivialization of ideas and images towards the universal. He will always be remembered for his passionate odyssey in making the beautiful a core part of his life, doing it purely out of love while drawing us along in the process.

While Buster the cat curled asleep in the basket beside Christopher's hospital bed at home, we had our last visit on the afternoon on December 16th. He looked at the unbudding of his fresh pink roses as I read an artist's letter from NYC detailing the Matisse exhibit. He asked for his glasses, and as I turned the pages of the Matisse catalog, he praised his favorite works while pointing out, in his opinion, the less successful pieces. And on that last afternoon, he tentatively expressed his misgivings about visiting the Matisse show, *impatient for Gina to bring a canvas so he could again work from his bed. After I massaged his hand, I kissed him on the forehead and slipped out, glad that he had seen the Christmas tree downstairs."*

** Footnote - My last visit with Christopher was on the night of the Dec.16th. He was weak and tired but excited about the art discussion he had enjoyed that day with Caroline. He also mentioned how he was still hopeful of going to see the Matisse exhibit. I gathered his dirty laundry to take to my house. I had tried to help in this way for some time, because Matthew had his hands full with caring for Christopher. Christopher was worried about me having to do his laundry and worrying about me working too much. As always, the protective brother was worrying about me. I kissed him, as I always did, on the cheek and told him I would see him the next day.

From Matthew's Eulogy

"It's probably just as well that most of you did not witness the final stages of Christopher's illness: God knows it was very hard to take for those of us who did. But Christopher always tried to make it easier for us and for the small army of medical professionals who worked on his care. Probably because he was still fighting his disease up to and including the day he died, no one around him ever gave up either."

Brushing Away The Tears

The next day, Thursday Dec.17, 1992, I got up and did Christopher's laundry. Strange things began happening that morning. I could hear a voice in my inner soul very plainly saying, "He won't need these things in heaven." I would then say out loud to myself, "Stop it! That is bad luck thinking." Later, I was wrapping some house shoes for him for Christmas and again I heard, "He won't need those in heaven," and on and on. About 11:30 a.m. or so, Matthew called me, frantically trying to find some equipment that had been misplaced having to do with the oxygen tank. He and Christopher had been to the doctor that day, and after getting Christopher up the steps, Christopher had collapsed. I didn't know where the equipment was, so I called Katy in Alabama to see if she remembered where it all was. I was overwhelmed with panic and felt bad as well for not being with them for that trip to the doctor. Finally, Matthew called me back and said he had called an ambulance, and they were taking him to the hospital and I could meet them there.

Looking back, I'm not sure why I didn't go to their house. I was in a total panic and I called Jeff, who told me not to drive in such a state, to stay there till he could get someone to drive me. Later, I found out he, my other roommates and my friend Tony Fowler had discussed what to do when the time came to help get me through my brother's death.

Brushing Away The Tears

A few minutes after I hung up the phone with Jeff, a calm came over me. I washed my face and got in my car and drove the long drive to Cedars Sinai. It was pouring rain and, yet when I was going by NBC in Burbank, the sun sent a strong beam down for a few moments and I said out loud, "Goodbye Sweet Christopher – you gave it all you had, and it is okay to let go now.". I wasn't crying or panicked. I was very calm as I drove.

I heard the most amazing songs on the radio on that drive. "No More Tears In Heaven" by Eric Clapton, "The Dance by Garth Brooks," Elton John's, "The Last Song," and most haunting of all, Bruce Springsteen's, "Streets of Philadelphia." I would briefly tell myself, "Don't think like that, he's not gone," But I knew with a certainty that I felt now (as I had never felt before) that he was truly at peace and that I would never see his sweet, loving face not ever again in this life.

I arrived at Cedars Sinai about 1:45 p.m. I went to the Emergency Room seeking my brother and Matthew. I was told that an ambulance had not brought them in yet. I went to the pay phone and called Matthew.

He said to me, "This is the worst thing I've ever had to tell anyone, and I'm so sorry it is on the phone; but Christopher died at 1:20.

Brushing Away The Tears

Please don't come over here, as the medics are still here, and I don't want you to see this. So please don't come and don't drive. I've called Jeff and he will send someone for you."

I immediately felt like a giant knife had been inserted into my stomach. I fell back into the phone bank screaming, "No, no!" and then asking if Matthew was okay. I remember thinking Christopher would want me to take care of Matthew. One of the ER employees came to my aid. Her last name was Wilson. Her name entered the small part of my brain that noticed anything except the overwhelming pain and grief that took over my being. She got a wheelchair for me. I briefly passed out. She talked to me and others hugged me and tried to console me. They wheeled me into a corner. Jeff called, and somehow they got the phone to me. He immediately told me Tony was on his way to drive me home. (I found out later they had all agreed on Tony because he and I were so close and he had been through something similar with his sister.) And Jeff told me how he had already talked with my parents and made arrangements for them to come to L.A. the next day. It is strange, but I didn't really want to talk to my parents in those first few hours. I guess it was because I didn't think I could handle any more pain than I already felt.

Tony arrived. We had a rough ride home, because Tony was not very familiar with driving a manual shift car. There was an eerie silence when I arrived at our house in Burbank. No one was there, and Tony stayed with me until Brian came home. Jeff didn't get home until much later because he was making arrangements, and I don't think he could bear to see me during those first few hours. His constant strength for me in handling all the daily details of living and helping my parents was invaluable. I was so blessed to have so many friends who were able to help me in their own unique ways.

GOD WILL SHOW ME THE WAY

Mom's Journal Entries

December 17, 1992 (before Christopher died)

Another day started with lots of tears. All I want to do is cry, but I have to go on.

Friday December 18, 1992 at the Houston airport

It happened.

My son is gone. My heart is at the bursting point. Nothing will ever be the same again. A part of me and Babe is gone forever. We're sitting in the Houston airport waiting to get to L.A. and to Deb. My soul aches for her. How can I make it better for her? Surely, God will show me a way.

A few hours after I got home, I finally got up enough courage to call Mom and Dad. It was so hard, and I don't remember a lot except Mom kept telling me that she would be with me the next day and there was a lot of crying. Friends called and I took comfort from those calls and in having my Los Angeles family around. Jeff finally came home, and he stayed with me for hours in my room. My dog, Max, was also a great comfort. My brother had paid for us to get Max at the animal shelter a few months after I moved to Los Angeles. He knew how much I missed having a dog.

The night was excruciatingly long. I woke up about 3:30 a.m. and called my brothers in Alabama. With the time difference it was 5:30a.m.and I knew they would most likely be awake. I cried and cried to them. Glenn was composing the local obit for the paper. I didn't have the will or the ability to do anything about arrangements. I was frozen in the grief. My usual desire to take control had vanished. Matthew, after weeks of having a difficult time coping, was able to take care of the necessary details that one must attend to when someone has died. He picked me up the day after Christopher died, and we went to the funeral home to make the arrangements. Christopher left a will that specified his desire to be cremated.

Mom's Journal Entry

December 22, 1992

We're in the air flying towards Nashville. I feel like I've left a part of myself behind. At least Debbie will be home tonight with us. I want to get somewhere that I can scream out my anger. Christopher was too young to die. It's hard to comprehend. Nothing left to feel and see, only his things. I would have liked to have seen him one last time, even though I know how cold in death he would have been. My family circle has been broken, a link gone forever. He's been dead since Thursday, but each day seems harder. I feel like I'm dreaming and will wake up and this nightmare will be over. I missed him so much when we got to his place Friday night. I know I have to be strong for Debbie and Babe. Tommy and Glenn too. I remember him as my little boy, especially since he has been sick. I wish Christmas was over. How will I ever get through it and all the people coming by and calling?

**Footnote - The following is an excerpt from the letter to Christopher that was the summary Matthew wrote to submit with the Quilt to the NAMES Project, which is the AIDS Quilt Organization.

Brushing Away The Tears

Matthew did such a wonderful job of verbalizing Christopher's story.

"It was December 15, 1992. Two days before you died. You asked the doctor if he would approve our going ahead with plans to visit the Matisse retrospective in New York. We were scheduled to leave in ten days. The doctor, glancing at me with a blank expression, assured you that it would be possible, provided things continued to go well. I remember watching the doctor's face as he spoke and knowing that was one trip we'd never make, but just like you, unwilling to give up the dream.

December 17, 1992 - The last day of your life. I've relived it in my mind thousands of times in minute detail. I remember what a struggle it was to dress you for your radiology appointment in Beverly Hills, how you had no energy at all, how I tried to convince you to cancel the appointment, how you refused. I remember how difficult it was to get your wheelchair down the steep thirty steps from our house to the street. Putting your sunglasses on to shield your dilated pupils, those soft blue eyes mostly just a memory now. When you arrived, you needed to go to the rest room. I remember your labored breathing as we struggled together to make you more comfortable, your distended abdomen a souvenir of your last desperate surgery a month earlier.

Brushing Away The Tears

The attendant finished the test, told us you could get dressed and left the room. You stood up unsteadily and immediately collapsed forward into my arms. For a moment, I thought you had gone, but then again I heard the wheezing, comforting sound of your breath. No one was around, so somehow I got you back into the wheelchair myself. Suddenly I was in a panic to get you of there. You were sitting semi-erect in the chair, unable or unwilling to talk. I wheeled you out of the building and back to the car, waiting in a parking structure about a block away. By then, you seemed to have recovered a bit and helped me get you into the front seat, your portable IV pump filling your veins with dilaudid, ensuring (or so I hoped) you had no pain. I got behind the wheel and thought, for the very first time, that all this had at last become too much for me.

You were almost yourself again on the way home, and we had our last conversation. As you had so often when you were healthy, you thought of a better route than the one I was taking and naturally I acquiesced. I wanted to lighten the mood and asked if you wanted to take the "scenic route." You said you were too tired for that, in a voice that made me believe it.

I kept all of your paintings. But if the house burns down tonight, it will be your final self-portrait I'll carry out from the flames. It was the first of two you were planning, to be called "Illness" It's successor, you were confident enough to declare, was to be "Recovery." And in it, you abandoned for the first time your quest for external beauty and color and instead embraced the stark reality within you in all its shades of grey and accents of blood red. You painted yourself nude, emaciated, sitting cross-legged, your torso wrapped in barbed wire. One half of the background was black, on the other half a small window of blue through cloudy sky, as if to balance or even deny the terror in your eyes.

The first thing I remember doing after you died is taking that painting down from its place of honor in the living room. Your body was still in the house, in fact still lying on the sofa in the same room, where you expired an hour or so after our return that day.

I'll never forget the talk we had one afternoon earlier that year, as you were working on the self-portrait. You said you had showed it to your mother, who was in town visiting. She had hated it, understandably enough given the subject matter. An so you had spent an impossible morning trying to lighten it up, make it more palatable, finally throwing your brush down onto the floor in frustration. 'I can't make this pretty, no matter how I try,' you said.

From the beginning, whenever you caught a cold or had some minor ailment, you always said, 'I don't suffer well.' But you were wrong.

You were magnificent. You never gave up. Toward the end, you spent much of your precious energy protecting those around you by exuding confidence and optimism. And in turn, your family and I refused to let you discover just how frightened we were. Everyone tired to behave courageously, as if you would get well if only we just believed it was possible. And, who knows, maybe that helped keep you alive.

But we never really talked about death, and we never really said goodbye. I wonder if it somehow would have been easier for you if we could have acknowledged our fear and anger. If some sort of resolution was possible before your departure, the truth is we didn't achieve it. But that's not to overlook what we did achieve. You discovered who you really were, and so did I. You maximized the intensity and enjoyment of your life, and showed me how to do the same. When it became obvious that we were not going to be allowed to grow old together, we grew up together instead. And when it was time for you to leave, you did so peacefully, with your quality of life and dignity absolutely intact. So perhaps resolution should be reserved for finished products, not human beings like me, or you. As long as I have a memory, I will have access to your loving spirit and a chance to live as you did—embracing, changing, feeling, forgiving.

Brushing Away The Tears

Which means the story isn't really over, after all."

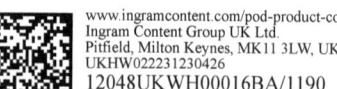
www.ingramcontent.com/pod-product-compliance
Ingram Content Group UK Ltd.
Pitfield, Milton Keynes, MK11 3LW, UK
UKHW022231230426
12048UKWH00016BA/1190